HEALTH UNLIMITED!

D0110924

HEALTH UNLIMITED!

Unleash Your Healing Power

by Alan M. Immerman, D.C.

32183

Naturegraph Publishers, Inc. Books for a Better World.

Library of Congress Cataloging in Publication Data

Immerman, Alan M., 1950—
  Health unlimited! Unleash your healing power.

  Includes bibliographical references.
  1. Health. 2. Healing. I. Title.
RA776.I55   1989   613   89-12695
ISBN 0-87961-202-9
ISBN 0-87961-203-7 (pbk.)

Naturegraph Publishers, Inc.
P.O. Box 1075
Happy Camp, CA 96039

Books for a better world

CONTENTS

NOTE: The use of the words "he, him, and his" refers to the traditional style of inclusiveness (he/she).

Section One

THE BASICS

INTRODUCTION

Are you tired of not feeling as well as you would like? Or do you feel pretty good but wish to feel great? Then this book is for you. Herein you will find the information you need to *take control of your health* and improve it dramatically.

Too many of us have relinquished control of our health. At the first sign of illness, we often rush off to the doctor who prescribes a pill with no explanation. We take the pill, feel better in a few days or weeks, then forget the whole incident. But this is rarely the smartest course to follow. To gain or maintain health, you must understand how you may be causing most of your illnesses, and then you must learn how to take action to build good health.

The purpose of this book is to teach the philosophy and methods needed to get well and stay well. It is exciting to realize that the body can actually heal itself without drugs and surgery. Most arthritics can become free of pain without medications. Heart patients can often avoid coronary bypass surgery. People suffering from chronic sinus problems, allergies, and asthmas can begin to feel great almost all the time. The list of health problems which can be resolved by simple lifestyle changes is quite long.

In practice there is nothing as satisfying as seeing a patient go from poor to good health. A person who has achieved good health is a wonder to behold, with shiny clear eyes, soft glowing skin, and a bouncy energetic step. A healthy person feels great most of the time, has lots of energy to share with his spouse and children, and has much vigor at work. Since physical health is impossible to achieve without mental health, a healthy person also has a positive mental attitude.

People will sometimes say that they are too busy to be concerned with their health. But this is a dangerous attitude. We must institute preventive health measures or we may suddenly find our supposedly firm foundation of good health ripped out from underneath us. Would you wait until your car died by the side of the road before you had the engine tuned-up? No. It is

« « « ◯ » » »

even more hazardous to take your health for granted because, if you loose your health, you may also lose the ability to work, take care of a family, and maintain a home. Maintaining health must be our *number one priority!*

There are those who think that they are "too far gone" to bother trying to improve their health. "I am hopeless," they say. But nothing could be further from the truth. If you are alive, you can improve your health! I have seen people in wretched shape who have dramaticaly improved the way they feel.

To be truly healthy, must you live like a monk in a cave with a multitude of sacrifices, denials, and limitations? No. The steps that we need to take to achieve better health are actually pleasant, comfortable, and fun. There are no major sacrifices. Life does not have to become serious, somber, and empty of fun.

A health-building lifestyle program does require some changes, but they are generally easy. For example, biting into a juicy sweet naval orange is delightful. Walking briskly around the block is exhilarating. Reducing the stress of life is relaxing. It is so wonderful to feel healthy that the minor sacrifices we need to make seem insignificant.

The information provided by this book will not make all drugs and surgical procedures obsolete. There are times when medical care will be necessary. With pneumonia, antibiotics may save lives; with cancer, chemotherapy can occasionally prolong life for years; with severe crippling hip arthritis, surgery may restore mobility. But most people choose drugs and surgery when they could have selected a safer and healthier alternative. With more information, an alternative path can usually be followed. I strongly suggest that you consult with a doctor who specializes in alternative methods to determine if you can recover your health through natural means.

The happy truth is that you can almost always feel better without using drugs and surgery. This book can serve as your guide. The first section, *The Basics,* will explain how your body works to heal itself when needed, and how you can listen to your body to determine what it needs. The second section, *How Trouble Develops,* will show you how illness is caused, and how it

« « « ○ » » »

can progress, for example, from a mild cold to the flu to arthritis to a heart attack.

The third section, *The Problems,* will discuss the most common and distressing illnesses from which people suffer. This section will apply the basic concepts of the first two sections to specific health problems.

The fourth section, *How To Unleash Your Body's Healing Powers,* will discuss the methods which you will need to use to build health. I will discuss nutrition, exercise, stress reduction, and the details of how to eat for health. You will find that you can eat healthfully and enjoy it.

In the back of the book you will find a bibliography. There are references to many articles in standard medical and scientific journals. These are important, because such articles are the foundation of modern scientific knowledge and truth. If you or your doctor want to know more, go to a medical library and read these articles.

The path to good health is easy to comprehend and simple to follow. The results are dramatic. Read on and learn how you can feel better than you ever imagined possible.

« « « 〇 » » »

LISTEN
TO YOUR BODY

When we hear about the newest high-tech computer, we are impressed. Imagine the capability of storing all the information found in a library within one small computer! Yet your brain is more sophisticated and complex than the most advanced computer ever imagined.

When we hear about the most recent development in heart surgery, we are impressed. Imagine the ability to replace a human heart with an artificial pump! Yet the ability of your heart to heal itself under the proper conditions is even more of a miracle than a heart transplant. No surgeon could ever do such a precision repair job. Unfortunately, however, most of us take the body for granted. We never take the time to become aware of how the body functions with great complexity every moment to sustain life.

Every moment that you are alive there is a virtual miracle happening within you. In the face of extremes of cold and hot temperatures, your body stays within a few degrees of normal. Every second, minute adjustments are made to maintain normal blood pressure, acidity, oxygen content, calcium levels, and literally thousands of other variables. The body's effort to maintain survival at the highest level of health possible every moment is enormous.

It is crucial that you understand and then develop great faith in the ability of your body to run its own affairs in the healthiest way possible. If you have this faith and you become sick, you will look to your body for the solution. If your body contains a computer more complex than has ever been imagined, if your body houses chemists more sophisticated than those found at the greatest universities on earth, then your body deserves more faith than you often give it.

One of the major purposes of this book is to teach you that your body can almost always heal itself without any outside help.

« « « ○ » » »

In fact, most of the symptoms of illnesses are direct evidence of healing activity. When you are sick, learn to listen to your body. If you can read the signals sent to you from your body, you will know how to respond in such a way as to help your body's healing activities.

Symptoms are produced by the body as messages to your conscious awareness. When you get pain, your body is telling you that there is trouble present. When you get other symptoms such as nausea, vomiting, diarrhea, coughing, sneezing, fever, fatigue, etc., your body is sending you a message. Always remember that symptoms are messages, not diseases. Don't be satisfied with health care approaches that solely eliminate symptoms. If you had a fire in your house, would you be satisfied with turning off the fire alarm as a solution? Of course not. But that is what we do when we deal with sickness by taking pills that only get rid of symptoms.

This book will help you learn to listen to your body. For instance, you will learn that the pain of inflammation is evidence of a healing process in action. You can actually help your body complete the healing process, instead of taking aspirin or something more powerful to suppress the inflammation.

You will learn that a cough is not a disease to be stopped, but rather a healing action. With a cough, your lungs are attempting to cleanse themselves. It is far better to help your lungs cleanse themselves than to take a drug to stop the cough, and you will herein learn how to help your lungs heal.

It has been said that the greatest doctor of all lives within your body. When you are sick, he tries to talk to you and tell you what to do. Once you learn how to listen to the doctor within you, and follow his advice, you will be on the path to feeling better than you ever dreamt possible.

« « « O » » »

WHAT IS HEALTH?

We all want to be healthy. Yet do we know what health is? Usually the answer is no. There are few classes on health in colleges, and none in medical schools. Research projects which study health are rare. As a result, most people do not know how to define "health."

Health is more than just feeling good. If you feel good one day, then are sick the next, you were not truly healthy when you felt good. It takes a long time to go from being healthy to having the symptoms of illness.

Dorland's Medical Dictionary says that health is "a state of optimal physical, mental, and social well-being, and not merely the absence of disease and infirmity." Clearly, feeling good does not always mean that one is healthy.

Our society, then, is suffering from a tragic lack of knowledge about health. Yet we have great expertise about disease. Scientists have categorized diseases, described diseases, studied the microscopic changes found in diseases, and researched cures for diseases. Yet, sadly, we are literally dying from the lack of knowledge about health.

But not everyone in our society is ignorant about health. I would like to introduce you to a true health revolution that began in the United States 150 years ago, and which continues to this day. Doctors of all types were, and still are, involved. Instead of curing disease, these doctors became interested in building health so that the body could have the vigor to heal itself. One of the doctors of this health revolution was Herbert Shelton. No one in history has been more clear about health and its requirements.

Dr. Shelton says that "health is the correct condition and action of all the vital powers and properties of the living body, and this necessitates the proper development and vigorous function of all the organs and tissues of the body and a close adherence to the laws and requirements of life. It is the normal or natural state of all organic existence and is always found where the laws and

« « « ◯ » » »

conditions of life are observed."

How do we build health? Dr. Shelton states that "the universal tendency of all organic existence, animal or vegetable, is towards health. Every organ and tissue in the living body is striving ceaselessly to maintain itself in as ideal a state as possible. To this law there is no known exception. Life strives always toward perfection. It is as natural to be healthy as it is to be born."

Dr. Shelton continues: "If the laws of life are complied with— if the conditions of healthy life are present—there is no power known to man which can prevent him from manifesting superb health. If these conditions are not present, the body must manifest as much health as the conditions present will permit. If health is already impaired, and the laws and conditions of healthy life are complied with, there is nothing that will prevent the living organism from returning to normal health, unless the destruction of vital parts or exhaustion of vital power have progressed beyond the body's power of repair and recuperation."

So, health is the normal condition of life when one carefully fulfills the requirements of life. Health is a state of optimal physical and mental functioning, not merely the absence of symptoms.

How can we know if we are healthy? Most people will say that if they feel good, then they are healthy. But this can be a dangerous error. Mayor Richard Daley of Chicago felt robust and vigorous at the time of a thorough physical examination in December, 1976. In the exam, doctors checked his height and weight, blood pressure and pulse; listened to his heart, lungs, and abdomen; looked at his eyes, ears, nose, and throat; performed extensive analysis of blood and urine; checked the heart with an electrocardiogram; and etc.

When the test results were studied, Mayor Daley was given a "clean bill of health." This was no surprise to him since he was feeling so good.

But a big surprise came one week later when Daley dropped dead of a massive heart attack! Is it possible that he could have gone from good health to fatal heart disease in one week? No. Mayor Daley was in terrible health when he had his complete

« « « ◯ » » »

examination, but there were no symptoms at that time. Heart disease must develop for many years before a fatal heart attack will occur. So even with a thorough examination and a sense of "feeling good," you cannot be sure that you are healthy.

Examining someone for symptoms or signs of disease is not a reliable way to determine if good health exists. A thorough examination is valuable, but beyond that the patient should have a complete analysis of his lifestyle habits. If the exam turns up no apparent problems, but the patient eats mainly greasy meats and drinks only sugary soda pop, we can conclude that good health is not present. If the person says he feels good, yet he never exercises or rests sufficiently, and he is under too much stress, good health is not present.

Because of the confusion over the meaning of the word "health," most people believe that by suppressing symptoms of disease they will restore health. We believe that taking an aspirin will cure a headache, that laxatives will cure constipation, that motrin will cure arthritis. Yet these drugs no more cure disease than turning off a fire alarm will "cure" a fire! *The symptom is not the disease.*

Most people take better care of their automobiles than of themselves. We do not wait for the car to break down before getting a tuneup. After 12,000 miles, we give the car a tuneup even if it is running smoothly. But with the body, we do nothing to improve the level of health until there is a breakdown. It is crucial to take steps to safeguard health even if we feel good. When ill, we must learn to help the body heal itself (extinguish the fire) and not just hide the symptoms of illness (turn off the fire alarm).

We do not live in a world of healthy people. The statistics of cancer, heart disease, diabetes, strokes, arthritis, and other chronic diseases are alarming. The incidence of the common cold, flu, bronchitis, pneumonia, sinusitis, and other acute diseases is appalling. We frequently hear that the average lifespan in the United States is increasing all the time, and that this proves that we have a country of healthy people. But we don't hear that the reason for the longer average lifespan is improved sanitation

« « « ○ » » »

which has resulted in a lower death rate for children and young adults. In middle age, the number of years that one can expect to live has changed very little in this century. We have a long way to go before we can say that America is a land of healthy people.

Fortunately, however, our society is moving in a healthward direction. People are trying to improve their diet, exercise more often, and reduce their stress. Many are learning that *good health is a matter of choice, not chance.* We can each choose to live more healthfully, and thereby become more healthy. Good health only results from healthful living, not symptomatic cures. You can learn to build health in the true meaning of the word, and this investment of time and energy will pay off better than any other you might make.

« « « ○ » » »

HEALTH
PHILOSOPHY

What is health philosophy? *Webster's Dictionary* says that health philosophy is a study of the general principles and laws which underlie all knowledge and reality of health. If we desire to build and maintain health, we must have a clear understanding of health philosophy. It is not sufficient to have a working knowledge of the details of healthful living. We need to understand the principles which underlie knowledge of health, or our commitment to healthful living practices may falter at a time of crisis. A clear health philosophy is the strong foundation upon which we will build a sturdy structure of health.

Must health philosophy be so complicated that only doctors can understand it? Absolutely not. The average person can easily understand the basics. Common sense is all that is needed. College education is totally unnecessary.

Some people do not want to be mentally involved with their health. They prefer to go about the tasks of daily living without thinking about the requirements of health or the causes of disease. If a symptom such as pain suddenly appears, they wish to go to a doctor who will "cure" them with little discussion. They do not want to know the details: the cause of the pain, the mechanics of the problem which manifested as pain, the way in which the alleged "cure" will solve the problem, and what will be necessary in the future to prevent a recurrence. They want a doctor who will make all the decisions without sharing any of his thinking.

But the type of person just described is fortunately becoming rare. Today most people want to know what is going on when sickness appears. They want to know how the problem was caused, what is going wrong inside the body, and how they can recover good health and prevent a recurrence. Such people will not tolerate the type of doctor who gets angry when he is asked too many questions. Many people would fire a doctor who, when

« « « ◯ » » »

asked about the details of an illness, would say "if you want to know so much, go to medical school!"

Every person has a fundamental need and right to secure knowledge about the requirements of health and the causes of illness. Never settle for less than a clear understanding of these issues. If you truly desire to take control of your health and become as full of vitality and vigor as possible, you must understand the basics of health philosophy.

Rule number one: *the foundation of health philosophy is that healing is a process accomplished by the body, and only by the body.* We live in a world of supposed cures. One pill will cure headache, another an upset stomach. One will cure a skin disease, another a sore throat.

But external substances cannot exert curative actions on the body. Chemical drugs which are ingested are inert and lifeless and therefore cannot act. When such substances are taken, the body acts on them. In our confusion, we usually say that the drug acted on the body and the body reacted. But this is impossible: a lifeless drug cannot act. Only a living being like the body can act.

So when we swallow a foreign chemical like a drug, the body will act on the drug. The science of pharmacology teaches that one of two things happens when a drug is ingested: the body will either speed up or slow down the pace of a normal activity. When either of these two changes takes place, the sick person who took the drug will feel different. But it is crucial to understand that this does not mean that a cure has been produced. All that results is a change in symptoms, not a resolution of the cause of the symptoms.

The body actions that truly heal the cause of the symptoms are completely different from the body actions that follow the ingestion of a drug. Health problems cannot be cured by swallowing foreign chemicals. The body is the only source of healing. Fortunately, when an illness develops, the body will automatically and spontaneously take steps to heal itself. Though we may feel better when we take drugs, our health status has not really improved.

Let's consider some examples. It is common for a person

« « « ◯ » » »

suffering from constipation to take a laxative. The laxative is a powerful chemical irritant, so irritating that when it finds its way into the intestine, the body will feel so insulted that it will vigorously eliminate the irritant along with all the intestinal contents. Would it be accurate to say that the laxative cured the constipation? No. The constipation developed because the intestine had been overworked and exhausted. The laxative did not make the intestine stronger or healthier in any way. In fact, since the chemical irritation of the laxative provoked the exhausted intestine to work very hard, the problem of constipation will be more severe following the use of the laxative. The intestine will be weaker, not stronger.

Patients with heart failure often take digitalis. After the patient swallows this drug, the heart will suddenly begin to beat with great strength. Is the heart failure cured? No. The heart had failed due to exhaustion, and digitalis cannot recharge the heart. Imagine a farmer using a horse to plow his field. At the end of the day, the horse is exhausted and lies down in the field. The farmer wants to finish the plowing, so he whips his horse into action. The horse gets up and finishes the task of plowing.

Did the whipping strengthen the horse? It may seem so, since the job did get finished. But no whip can strengthen a horse. More work may get done by using a whip, but the exhausted horse will only get more exhausted and weak. Months and years of such treatment will reduce the overall amount of work which the horse will be able to accomplish.

Taking digitalis for a weak heart is the same as whipping a tired horse in the field. The whip does not strengthen the horse, nor does the digitalis strengthen the heart.

What if a person has a headache and takes an aspirin? The pain will disappear, but was the problem cured? No. The pain arose from a troubled area of the body, much like a warning light comes on in a car if the oil level is too low. The aspirin only removed the awareness of the problem, not the problem itself. No one would disconnect the oil warning light instead of adding oil when the alert light went on, but some people do this every day with their headaches.

« « « ◯ » » »

Earlier I said that pharmacology teaches that the use of drugs can only result in an increase or decrease of the pace of normal body actions. Laxatives and digitalis result in an increase in intestinal and heart activity, respectively. Aspirin results in a decrease in the function of the nerves which convey the message of pain from a troubled area of the body to the center in the brain which registers pain. The use of each of these drugs will make a person feel better. But, such drug use will not produce one bit of healing.

Pneumonia and other infections may seen to be exceptions to the rule that drugs do not cure diseases. However, upon deeper analysis, we find that the rule holds true. Antibiotics will destroy the bacteria involved with the infection, but they will not cure the cause of infections which is lowered body resistance. Infections sometimes are so severe that antibiotics are needed, but these drugs do not improve resistance to infections, and therefore, are not true cures. Only the body itself can work to increase health and resistance to the point where infections are rare.

Instead of looking for cures, we should work to support the body's healing process. This can be done by providing the body with the normal raw materials of life, and by not obstructing the healing process. Specifically, healthy food must be eaten in proper amounts, exercise should be of the right type and frequency, rest must be sufficient, stress must not be excessive, pure air and water should be sought after, and the body should be exposed to natural sunlight for the proper amount of time.

Good health is a product of healthful living, not cures. Though healthful living of itself cures nothing, it unleashes the body's healing power which can do more than all the doctors in the world combined. Never underestimate this strength.

Rule number two: *the body almost always acts in its own best interests.* When a person becomes acutely ill, many uncomfortable and distressing symptoms develop: vomiting, coughing, fever, sneezing, diarrhea, pain, muscle tension, etc. Except in rare instances, these symptoms arise from the vigorous expression of the healing power. When the body eliminates waste material from

« « « ◯ » » »

the intestines or lungs, it is because the brain determined that health would be improved by such elimination. Attempting to suppress such symptoms with drugs makes one sicker, not healthier. There are rare exceptions, such as pneumonia, but this rule holds true 99% of the time.

Rule number three: *the short term effect is opposite to the long term effect.* A cup of coffee apparently increases energy; in fact, the long term effect is more fatigue. Coffee gives the body no energy; it occasions the release of stored energy, thereby further depleting the body.

This rule has been called the law of stimulation. Apparent stimulants actually weaken the body. Laxatives weaken an exhausted intestine, and digitalis weakens a worn-out heart. The short term effect of greater intestinal and heart activity leads to the long term effect of increased weakness and exhaustion. No external substance can give energy to the body. The energy output which follows the use of coffee, laxatives, and digitalis comes from the body, not the drug. Foods, as opposed to drugs, do not stimulate the body. Rather, they provide the body with the proper raw materials from which the body can create energy.

The flu is another example of the short term effect being the opposite of the long term effect. One feels terrible while the lungs and sinuses discharge large amounts of waste material. The intestines may eject material from both ends with vomiting and diarrhea. The short term feeling is one of severe illness. Yet the long term effect is better health. The flu is a time of vigorous elimination of waste material. When the body harbors less of the waste material that had accumulated for months, the overall health level will be greater. (See chapters on Toxemia and Infectious Diseases for a deeper understanding of the flu.)

Rule number four: *drugs and surgery should only be used as a last resort.* Drugs are powerful chemicals all of which have many negative side effects. One hundred changes in body function may follow the use of a drug. Of these, one may be desirable and 99 undesirable. The 99 unwanted changes are called the side effects.

Because of the side effects, a healthy person who takes a drug will become sick. Yet we expect that the same drug will produce

« « « ◯ » » »

health in a sick person. This is impossible; drugs do not build health, they suppress symptoms, and at great cost. Turning off the fire alarm (the symptom) with a drug will not extinguish the fire (the cause of the symptom). Drugs can save lives in some cases, but probably 90% of the time drugs are given, they produce more harm than good.

These are the basics of health philosophy, the general principles and laws which underlie all knowledge and reality of health. Those who do not understand them will remain confused with no direction and poor health. But it is exciting to realize that each of us can learn health philosophy, take control of our health, and feel much better than we ever imagined possible.

« « « O » » »

Section Two

HOW TROUBLE DEVELOPS

TOXEMIA

In the 20th century, the word "toxemia" is not commonly used when people discuss health and disease. This is a situation that needs to be changed because many health problems stem from toxemia.

Toxemia results from accumulation in the body of chemical substances which are toxic in any amount, or of substances which are non-toxic in normal amounts but toxic when in excess. When a chemical is toxic, it will inflict damage on the body.

Chemicals which are toxic when present in any amount are arsenic, lead, lye, mercury, asbestos, botulism poison, etc. These chemicals will cause severe illnesses which may even be fatal. Lead poisoning, for instance, can result from eating chips of paint. It will often cause severe brain damage.

Chemicals which are non-toxic when present in normal amounts but toxic when present in excess also may cause toxemia. To understand the cause of toxemia from a build-up of normal body chemicals, picture the body as a funnel. Foods are poured in the larger opening of the funnel. The body must burn, utilize, or eliminate what is ingested. But the body has only a limited capacity to process foods as represented by the smaller end of the funnel.

Between the top and bottom of the funnel, the body makes hundreds of changes in the food. Chemical A is converted to chemical B which is converted into chemical C, then D, then E, etc. When an excess of food is ingested, the funnel gets overloaded and there is a backup. The result is a great increase in the amounts of all body chemicals, A to Z. These chemicals are called intermediary metabolites and many are known to be toxic when present in excessive amounts. Such metabolites frequently are the cause of disease.

A major cause of aging is the development of crosslinkages between protein molecules. Crosslinkages cause joint stiffness and wrinkling in later life. Aging in the form of crosslinkages

« « « O » » »

represents an overall weakening and deterioration of the body. Excessive amounts of intermediary metabolites cause cross-linkages. Biochemists are very familiar with some of these chemicals, such as pyruvic acid, citric acid, malic acid, fumaric acid, and alpha ketoglutaric acid. Overeating causes a buildup of such chemicals and this results in damage to the body. Hundreds of studies have shown that eating a relatively small amount of food will delay aging. The body is able to completely process all of the food when less is eaten so there is no buildup of the intermediary metabolites which speed up the aging process.

There are many other normal body chemicals which are known to cause disease when present in excessive amounts. One of the most famous is cholesterol. It is needed to form chemicals which aid in the digestion and absorption of fats, for the manufacture of many hormones which regulate body function, and for the construction of the membranes which enclose all body cells. Dietary sources of cholesterol are meats, dairy products, and eggs. If excessive amounts of these foods are eaten, the blood cholesterol level will soar, and the risk of a heart attack or stroke will increase.

Triglycerides are the fats in our diet and bloodstream. They are an important source of energy for the body. Triglycerides come from the saturated fats in animal foods, the unsaturated fats in vegetable foods, and from sugars and starches via conversion in the liver. An elevated triglyceride level makes the blood cells become sticky and clump together. This reduces blood flow and can cause a heart attack, stroke, or other serious problem.

Uric acid is another chemical which is normally present in the bloodstream. It comes from eating meats, drinking alcohol, breakdown of body tissue, and production within the body. High levels of uric acid in the bloodstream will cause a serious form of arthritis called gout.

Glucose is blood sugar. It comes from the breakdown of starch and sugar, or conversion from fat and protein. An elevated level of glucose, as is found in diabetes, will damage the blood vessels, nervous system, muscles, and eyes. This damage can cause a heart attack, stroke, numbness, weakness, impotence,

« « « ◯ » » »

cataracts, and blindness.

Homocysteine is a chemical that comes from the breakdown of protein. If blood levels of homocysteine become too high from eating too much protein, the walls of blood vessels will be irritated. Such irritation leads to the buildup of fat deposits which can cause a heart attack or stroke.

The concept of toxemia was developed in the early 20th century by John H. Tilden, M.D. He stated that stress from daily habits or from the environment will excessively strain the body. This strain will affect both the mind and body and lead to overall exhaustion which Tilden called enervation. When enervation develops, the body becomes too weak to efficiently eliminate toxins of any type through the liver, lungs, intestines, kidneys, or skin.

Inefficient elimination leads to retention of toxins. When there is an excessive accumulation of normal or abnormal chemicals, the condition is called toxemia.

A continual rise in toxin levels will inevitably exceed the body's level of tolerance. When the point of intolerance is reached, the body will attempt to eliminate the toxins. Symptoms of such elimination include sneezing, coughing, vomiting, diarrhea, skin secretions, and dark urine. These symptoms are evidence of a health-building process. They should be welcomed as signs of vigorous healing.

If the body has been overwhelmed for too many years with toxins, it may not have the strength to do an effective job of cleansing and elimination. When toxins are present for a long time, chronic illnesses will develop. An example is heart disease from a buildup of cholesterol.

Advanced toxemia will irritate all areas of the body. Because of heredity, or the past history of health problems, one area of the body will be weaker than other areas. This weaker area will show signs of disease first. Therefore the same toxins may cause a lung problem in one person but a kidney problem in another.

Dr. Tilden in his research discovered many causes of enervation and toxemia. Nutritional causes include overeating, eating the wrong foods, vitamin and mineral deficiences, use of

« « « ◯ » » »

coffee, tea, or alcohol. Emotional causes include worry, jealousy, rage, and fear. Miscellaneous causes include toxins produced by bacteria, an uncongenial environment, injuries, postural tension, physical defects, physical excesses, and the unpoised state.

The solution for toxemia is to support the body as it attempts to solve the problem. The body does not need to be cleansed by laxatives, enemas, or similar measures since it is fully capable of cleansing itself. When the body tries to eliminate toxins through coughing, diarrhea, and other means of elimination, we should not fight against this process. Taking drugs to stop the mucous flow of a cold or to stop diarrhea will stop toxin elimination.

The only time to take drugs is when the intensity of the cleansing process is too great. For instance, a child with severe diarrhea lasting for more than two days can become dehydrated and die without drugs. An elderly patient with a severe cough from pneumonia could also die without drugs. But these are the rare exceptions. In most cases it is safe to weather the storm of a cleansing crisis without taking drugs. It is best to have a knowledgeable doctor supervising your care.

When the body is permitted to complete the elimination it has begun, toxins will not remain locked up in the body. In this way, the chronic illnesses which result from long-lasting toxemia will be less likely to develop, or less severe in intensity when they do occur.

« « « ◯ » » »

INFLAMMATION

Arthritis, gastritis, tonsillitis, and bronchitis are diseases of different body regions. Yet they are more alike than different since all are inflammatory conditions. Any disease name which ends in "itis" is an inflammation.

Whether it is found in the joints or the throat or elsewhere, inflammation has the same purpose and result. The list of inflammatory diseases is quite long since this process can occur in any area of the body. Naming the condition requires using the name of the tissue and adding "itis" to the end. "Arth" means joint, so arthritis is inflammation of a joint. "Gastric" means stomach, so gastritis is inflammation of the stomach.

From the way in which inflammatory conditions are named, it would seem that they are all different diseases. For instance, bronchitis is obviously not identical to tonsillitis. But because the basic process which occurs in the tissue is identical wherever it is found, conditions of inflammation are the same throughout the body. The causes are the same, the mechanics are the same, and the results are the same. When you understand the nature of inflammation in a joint, you understand the nature of inflammation in the intestine, pancreas, brain, or wherever it occurs.

What is inflammation? Robbins' *Pathologic Basis of Disease,* a top medical textbook, says that inflammation is the local reaction of tissue to injury. Inflammation has been understood for centuries. In 1793 a Scottish surgeon wrote what is now considered obvious: inflammation is not a disease but a response by the body that has a health-building effect.

Robbins' says that inflammation "serves to destroy, dilute, or wall-off the injurious agent and the tissue cells that it may have destroyed. In turn, the inflammatory response sets into motion a complex series of events which, as far as possible, heal and reconstitute the damaged tissue... Without inflammation, bacterial infections would go unchecked, wounds would never heal, and injured tissues and organs might remain permanent festering

« « « ◯ » » »

defects."

Inflammation is therefore, a healing activity which is initiated by the body when the need is present. For example, consider the case of a splinter that became lodged in the skin. The splinter is clearly an injurious agent. Nerves to the skin register the presence of the splinter and alert the brain. As a result, the brain activates the inflammatory process to destroy the splinter. Blood will be rushed to the area to provide white blood cells which release chemicals to digest the splinter. The extra blood causes the skin to become reddened and swollen. The area will feel hot and painful. Within a few hours or days, the splinter will be dissolved.

Inflammation can only arise when there is a need for it in the form of some agent which is harmful to the body. The activities of inflammation are basically the same wherever they occur. The characteristics which distinguish inflammation in one area of the body from the same process in a different area result from the nature of the involved tissue and the degree of intensity of the inflammation.

It is clear that inflammation is a health-building process, initiated only when the brain perceives a need for such action. Because inflammatory diseases are commonplace, it is crucial to understand the basic nature of inflammation and to follow a rational path to resolve the problem. With a splinter, we should first attempt removal with sterile tweezers and needle. If the splinter is too deep we should let the body destroy it from within by the actions of inflammation.

Most of the inflammatory conditons are internal. Since we cannot remove irritants from joints with tweezers, we must depend upon the effectiveness of the inflammatory process.

Inside the body, the injurious agent which the body tries to destroy with inflammation is usually a chemical toxin. Toxemia, the presence of irritating toxins in the body, is extremely common (see chapter on toxemia). Toxins are found in the bloodstream, in the tissue spaces between cells, and within cells. When the body becomes excessively irritated by the toxins, it will turn on the inflammatory process.

The best way to deal with an inflammatory disease is to help it

« « « ◯ » » »

along. Because inflammation is the body's chosen form of treatment for toxemia, we do not need to treat toxemia with any other methods. The best course to follow is one of complete rest. With proper rest, we do nothing which interferes with the inflammatory process.

Complete rest involves resting the digestive system by eating a minimal amount of food and/or fasting, resting the body by staying home from work and not exercising, and resting the mind by not worrying and fretting. When we eat less, the body will live on non-essential substances within the system. The first to be burned for energy will be the accumulated toxins. Most of the toxins are normal body chemicals which, because they are present in excessive amounts, have a toxic effect. Conserving energy by resting the body and mind allows the body to direct all available energies to the healing process.

In actual practice these measures are quite effective. Arthritis, bronchitis, sinusitis, colitis, gastritis, myositis, and many other inflammatory conditions resolve rapidly under the "complete rest" system of management. The chances of success, and the degree of safety, are greatly increased when one is supervised by a doctor familiar with these methods.

How do most doctors deal with inflammatory diseases such as arthritis and gastritis? Based on the fact that inflammation is a health-building process, you might assume that no doctor would ever try to halt this healing activity. But unfortunately you would be wrong. An incredible misunderstanding has developed: many doctors believe that the inflammation, not the cause of the inflammation, is the problem. Therefore an attack is made on the inflammatory process, not on the injurious agent which caused the inflammation.

Why the attack on inflammation? Because the symptoms of inflammation can be alarming. There can be a disturbing amount of pain, swelling, redness, heat, and disability associated with inflammation. Unfortunately, these symptoms are often regarded as the disease itself. The pain of inflammation, therefore, is treated as if it were the disease, instead of evidence of the body's effort to destroy the disease-producing agent.

« « « ◯ » » »

This is the rationale behind modern treatment of inflammatory diseases. Tons of anti-inflammatory drugs are swallowed by sick people every day. Examples of such drugs are cortisone, aspirin, naprosyn, and motrin. There are many others, with new ones appearing on the market every year.

Doctors mistakenly believe that the pain is the disease, not the symptom of the disease, so when the pain is gone the disease is thought to be cured. But stopping the inflammatory process is no more sensible than turning off a fire alarm instead of extinguishing the fire.

When the body becomes excessively loaded with toxins, the brain will initiate a series of measures to expel and destroy toxins. Sneezing, coughing, diarrhea, vomiting, and a runny nose are all forms of elimination. The inflammatory process is designed to destroy toxins within the body. Such healing activities should not be suppressed with drugs. Rather, they should be supported with proper lifestyle changes.

When inflammation is stopped by improper treatment, the toxins which the body was trying to eliminate will remain locked up in the bloodstream and tissues. The chronic toxemia which results will cause diseases which can be quite severe such as disabling arthritis and life-threatening heart disease.

We should respect the inherent wisdom of inflammation and not attempt to halt this process. In almost every case of inflammatory disease, the body, if properly supported, will complete the healing inflammatory activity it initiated and restore the organ or tissue to good health.

If you learn to cooperate with your body when it is trying to heal itself, you will develop a higher level of health than you have ever imagined possible. Find a doctor who understands that inflammation is good for you, and follow the path to true health.

« « « ◯ » » »

PROGRESSION OF PATHOLOGY

What is pathology? *Dorland's Medical Dictionary* defines pathology as the "structural and functional changes in tissues and organs of the body which cause or are caused by disease." A pathological condition of the body occurs when the body or one of its parts is not functioning normally and healthfully.

In the last two chapters we discussed toxemia and inflammation. The purpose of this chapter is to connect toxemia with inflammation and discuss a model of disease which explains how one phase of pathology progresses to another phase.

In the chapter on toxemia we explored the concept of enervation. Enervation is a state of overall body fatigue and exhaustion. When the body is enervated it cannot perform its functions to the normal degree. Enervation is the result of overeating, eating the wrong foods, excessive stress, too little exercise, insufficient rest, etc.

The result of enervation is toxemia. If the causes of enervation are not halted, toxemia will develop. When the body is fatigued it will do an incomplete job of removing toxins. Therefore the toxins will accumulate. The pathological condition of enervation has progressed to the pathological condition of toxemia.

When toxemia is present, the toxic chemicals will irritate body tissues. Toxins accumulate in all areas of the body, including the bloodstream which bathes every body tissue. Each of us has certain areas in the body which are weaker than other areas. Usually this is determined by inheritance: if your parents have heart trouble, you will probably have a tendency to develop heart problems; if your parents have sinus trouble, you will probably have relatively sensitive sinuses; if your parents have stomach problems, you will probably have a stomach which is easy to

« « « O » » »

irritate.

Persistent toxemia will progress to the stage of irritation. When body tissues are chronically exposed to toxins they will become irritated.

When irritation is present for a prolonged period of time the body will initiate a healing effort to destroy the toxins which are responsible for the irritation. This healing effort is called inflammation. The body will rush white blood cells to the area of irritated tissue and these cells will release powerful enzymes to destroy the irritating toxins. Inflammation is a healthful activity.

Sometimes the body cannot do the job solely with inflammation as its main healing activity. If the inflammatory process cannot do the complete job of toxin destruction the body will initiate other activities to help. We call these activities "vicarious elimination."

Acts of vicarious elimination include vomiting, sneezing, diarrhea, coughing, discharge of mucous from the nose, and excretions of waste by the skin. We tend to look at these activities as destructive actions which must be suppressed by nose sprays, cough syrups, and other drugs. But these actions are initiated by the body to eliminate harmful toxins. The liver filters toxins out of the blood and then it discharges these through the bile ducts into the upper small intestine. If these toxins are sent "downstream," they will pass through and bathe the tissues of approximately 35 feet of intestine. The body may choose, therefore, to spare this large area of intestine from irritation and send the toxins "upstream" a few inches into the stomach. The body will then discharge these chemicals with vomiting.

When vomiting occurs it is because the body wishes to eliminate toxins which are present in the stomach and upper small intestine. The same is true with the other activities of vicarious elimination. When coughing occurs the lungs are trying to cleanse themselves. When diarrhea occurs the intestines are trying to unload waste materials.

Unfortunately, the symptoms of healing and cleansing are usually regarded as the disease itself. The pain of inflammation, the discomfort of vomiting and diarrhea, the irritation of coughing,

« « « ◯ » » »

the nuisance of a runny nose, these and all other symptoms of healing are often suppressed with drugs. Such suppression prevents the body from cleansing itself of irritating toxins. When the toxins remain in the body for a prolonged period of time the pathological state of vicarious elimination will progress to the pathological state of ulceration.

Prior to the onset of ulceration very few body tissues have been destroyed. Irritation, inflammation, and vicarious elimination do not involve any significant tissue destruction. But when irritating toxins are present for too long a period of time, tissue destruction will occur. Such tissue destruction is called ulceration.

With significant ulceration the body will be unable to build enough new cells to replace the ones which have been destroyed. To fill in where cells have been destroyed the body will produce scar tissue. An example is cirrhosis of the liver which occurs after large-scale liver destruction by alcohol. The pathological condition of ulceration has progressed to the pathological condition of scar tissue, also called fibrosis or induration.

Up to this point there has been a tremendous progression of pathology. The initial stage of enervation which can usually be corrected by simple dietary changes and extra rest has progressed to the stage of fibrosis where body tissues have been destroyed and cannot be replaced. If the causes of disease are not halted at this point, the pathology may progress to the final stage of cancer. Chronic irritation by toxins may finally disrupt normal cells so much that they will go "haywire" and become cancerous.

The eight stages of pathology described above are a hypothetical explanation of how disease is produced in the body. There may be cases where this explanation does not apply. However in most cases it will apply and it is extremely useful in understanding how the body works.

Let's consider an example. Alcohol is a toxin to the body. A person who drinks excessively will weaken his body, thereby producing the state of enervation.

Because alcohol is a powerful toxin its presence in the body will produce the pathological condition of toxemia. If such toxemia persists the stage of irritation will result.

« « « ◯ » » »

Imagine the lining of the stomach being exposed to the toxic impact of alcohol. Severe irritation will commonly result. If the irritation persists the body will attempt to protect itself with inflammation.

The process of inflammation is initiated by the body to destroy the toxic chemical alcohol. The stomach lining will become reddened as the body rushes more blood and defensive white blood cells to the area. The inflammatory process is quite painful so the person who drank too much alcohol will be aware of what he has done to himself.

If the inflammatory process cannot complete the cleansing the body will initiate the process of vicarious elimination. In the stomach this will take the form of vomiting. Those who have had too much to drink have experienced this displeasure when the stomach attempts to free itself of irritating toxins.

If the stomach is not able to protect itself from the toxin alcohol through the processes of inflammation and vicarious elimination, stomach cells will be destroyed. This is the pathological stage of ulceration. A stomach ulcer can be caused by excessive drinking.

When healing of a stomach ulcer occurs scar tissue is usually formed. The stomach cannot completely heal an ulcer with normal stomach cells. Scar tissue is used, constituting the stage of fibrosis.

If the irritation of the stomach continues past this point, severe derangement of stomach cells can occur and cancer cells may form. Cancer is the final and irreversible stage of pathology.

The theme of this book is that most diseases are the direct result of unhealthful lifestyle practices. Such practices first result in enervation. If they are continued the pathology will progress from enervation to toxemia, then to irritation, then inflammation, vicarious elimination, ulceration, fibrosis, and finally, cancer. Certainly there are exceptions to this concept of the progression of pathology, but, in most cases disease can be best understood utilizing this model. If we always remember the steps of this progression we will have a much more profound understanding of the causes and solutions to health problems.

« « « ◯ » » »

Section Three

THE PROBLEMS

HEART DISEASE & STROKES

Cardiovascular diseases, primarily heart attacks and strokes, are responsible for more deaths in the United States than any other illnesses, including cancer. The underlying cause of cardiovascular diseases is atherosclerosis, the buildup of fat in blood vessels. This buildup blocks the blood flow to the heart and brain, which starves these vital tissues of oxygen and causes cells to die. A heart attack occurs when heart muscle cells die and a stroke occurs when brain cells die.

Where does the fat come from that blocks the blood vessels? In the 1980s this question has been conclusively answered. Atherosclerosis comes primarily from eating the wrong foods, especially high cholesterol foods.

In 1977 the National Institute of Health (NIH) began a program of "consensus development." When there is a pressing issue at hand, the NIH will gather together a group of about a dozen experts who will analyze all the facts at hand and come to a group conclusion, or "consensus."

In 1984 the NIH held a consensus development conference to discuss the relationship of high cholesterol foods to a high blood cholesterol level and the effect of a high blood cholesterol level on the risk of cardiovascular disease. The group of experts concluded that a diet high in saturated fat and cholesterol will raise the blood cholesterol level. Also, an elevated blood cholesterol level will increase the risk of heart attacks and strokes.

The NIH experts strongly feel that all Americans should reduce their intake of saturated fat and cholesterol and that people at a high risk of developing cardiovascular disease should make drastic dietary changes. The foods which should be eaten in much smaller quantities than is usual in the U.S. are meat, eggs, and dairy products.

« « « O » » »

Incredibly, despite the strong evidence to the contrary, there are still some who claim that a high fat diet does not cause fat deposits in blood vessels and cardiovascular diseases. They will advise you to eat all the eggs and cheese you want without worrying about your heart. This advice is, however, totally irresponsible since scientists have definitely proven the connection between a high fat diet and heart disease. I suggest you follow the position advocated by 99.9% of all scientists, not the thinking of the .1% minority.

How common is atherosclerosis? It kills over 550,000 Americans each year so it must be quite common. In reading medical literature, I was startled to find out that atherosclerosis is frequently found, even in young people. In the Korean War autopsies were performed on 300 servicemen who died in action, average age 22. Significant amounts of fatty deposits were found in the blood vessels of over 77% of these young soldiers.

From this we can assume that the average American has potentially dangerous amounts of fat buildup in his blood vessels from a very early age onward.

Scientific evidence has proven that meat, eggs, and dairy products, due to their high saturated fat and cholesterol content, are the main culprits in heart disease. But scientists have also found that more fat will be deposited in blood vessels if the walls of the blood vessels have previously been irritated or injured.

One of the most common causes of such irritation is a high protein diet. American are known to eat three times more protein than they need (see chapter on protein). A diet excessively high in protein will increase the level of homocysteine in the bloodstream which will irritate the walls of blood vessels, causing fat to be deposited. Therefore a high protein diet must also be avoided.

Many people, by changing their diets, will be able to avoid fat accumulation in blood vessels. But what can be done if the fat deposits are already present? Will coronary bypass surgery be needed to remove the clogged blood vessels and install new ones? In most cases the answer is no because the body has a tremendous capability to remove fat deposits which have already formed.

« « « ◯ » » »

In the past, scientists thought that cholesterol in fat deposits could never be removed. Recently however, studies have proven that cholesterol is mobile and will frequently move into and out of deposits. Researchers have marked cholesterol in order to monitor its movements.

Usual sources of blood cholesterol are diet and production by the liver. When a person fasts and drinks only water, no cholesterol is ingested, but the blood cholesterol level will rise. Where does the increase come from? Scientists have concluded that it comes from the breakdown of deposits in blood vessels.

During World War II, when fatty foods were in short supply in Europe, the death rate from cardiovascular diseases dropped. Autopsies showed far less blood vessel fat deposits than expected. Researchers believe that the wartime low fat diet gave the body a chance to dissolve the fat deposits.

Autopsies on people who have died of "wasting" diseases such as cancer have also revealed far fewer deposits of fat than expected. Cancer patients are usually of normal weight or overweight before they lose many pounds in the months before death. With weight loss the body breaks down fat deposits in blood vessels.

In experiments with monkeys, the type of animal most similar to man, it has been proven that a high fat, high cholesterol diet will cause a buildup of fat in blood vessels. If the diet is then changed to one low in fat and cholesterol, the fat deposits will be broken down and eliminated.

Therefore we can conclude that it is scientifically proven that the body can break down fat deposits in blood vessels when given a chance. To accomplish this, you need to eat less high fat foods such as meat, eggs, cheese, milk, butter, mayonnaise, shortening, etc. Eat three to four times more of the low fat foods such as fruits, vegetables, and grains, (rice, bread, oats, etc.). Consider fasting, but only under supervision of an experienced doctor.

As is the case with all health problems, diet is not everything. Exercising sufficiently and reducing stress will also decrease the risk of cardiovascular diseases.

In England, researchers studied 16,882 male middle-aged

« « « ◯ » » »

executives. They found that the men who exercised vigorously on a regular basis had one-third the risk of heart disease of the men who did not exercise. In another study it was found that men who ran the most miles had the healthiest blood cholesterol levels. The speed was not as important as the distance run.

Many scientists have found that a high stress lifestyle will increase the risk of cardiovascular diseases. Those people who are more aggressive, hard-working, achievement-oriented, time-conscious, impatient, and irritable usually have a higher risk of heart attack than people who are better able to relax.

Heart attacks and strokes kill more Americans than any other diseases. Yet they can be prevented with a healthful diet, regular exercise, and sufficient relaxation. When fat deposits have already developed the body can eliminate them if a healthful diet is used. Treat your heart right and it will give you a full lifetime of vigorous, consistent service.

« « « ◯ » » »

HIGH BLOOD PRESSURE

The TV ad says: "High blood pressure afflicts millions of people. Don't assume that your blood pressure is normal. High blood pressure has no symptoms; it is a silent killer. If your pressure is high, you may not know it until a devastating heart attack, stroke, or kidney disease strikes. See your doctor regularly to have your blood pressure checked. And, if it is high, follow your doctor's recommendations and take your drugs religiously."

High blood pressure is extremely common. It is also dangerous. Even mildly high pressure increases the chance of a stroke, heart attack, and kidney disease. 140/90 is considered the upper limit of normal blood pressure. Yet the Insurance Company 1979 Build and Blood Pressure Study found that when the first number in the blood pressure equation is between 138 and 147, the risk of death from strokes, heart attacks, and kidney failure is 36% higher in men and 22% higher in women than when the reading is lower. When the second number is between 88 and 92, the risk of death is 38% higher in men and 33% higher in women. Therefore we should not feel safe with a blood pressure reading of 140/90, the upper limit of so-called normal. If the reading is higher than 140/90 the danger is even greater.

Drugs are the common remedy for high blood pressure. Just take the drugs the rest of your life and you'll be fine. Sounds simple, doesn't it? Yes, except for one fact: all blood pressure medications have serious side effects ranging from cancer (reserpine) to anemia and jaundice (diuril) to heart failure and mental depression and nausea (inderal). What a choice people are given! Choose between these side effects and a stroke!

Fortunately, however, you need not be caught between a rock and a hard place. There are many solutions for high blood pressure besides drugs.

« « « ◯ » » »

Ninety percent of all people with high blood pressure have what is called the "essential" type. This basically means that the cause is not known (Kidney disease has been ruled out). It is the essential type of high blood pressure that responds well to non-medical remedies. At least 16% of all Americans between ages 18 and 79 have essential high blood pressure. And in older age groups the incidence is 40%.

Many lifestyle changes will result in lower blood pressure. For instance, one medical doctor fasted 683 overweight people and reported his results in a scientific journal. At the start of the fast (water diet), 48% had high blood pressure. Yet within two to four days, it was "rare for the blood pressure not to be normal." Occasional fasting then is an excellent way to control blood pressure. It is safe if done under careful supervision: don't just drop your medication and fast at home. If a proper diet is eaten after a fast the blood pressure will remain lower.

What other lifestyle changes will lower blood pressure? First, salt must be eliminated from the diet. This includes salt added at the table, plus hidden salt found in most processed foods (cheese, butter, bread, pastries, etc.). Eat large amounts of high potassium foods (fruits and vegetables). This will help neutralize the harmful effects of sodium.

Second, eat fewer calories and reduce to thin body weight. It has been estimated that if obesity were controlled in the white population of the United States, the number of people with high blood pressure could be cut in half. Calorie intake and resultant body weight are probably even more important than salt intake. For instance, one study found that when obese patients ate a diet low in calories but average in salt content, 70% achieved normal blood pressure.

Third, exercise regularly. Again, scientific studies have proven that regular exercise will help control blood pressure. In one study, a group of men exercised intensely for about one-half hour two times per week under careful supervision. A significant drop in blood pressure was noted after six months. Another study used weekly exercise sessions lasting two hours. One hundred eighty-one sedentary middle-aged men did calisthenics, jogged, or played volleyball during a six month program. At the end of the experiment all participants, both those with and without high blood pressure, experienced a drop in pressure.

But, if you have been sedentary for years don't plunge into a five-mile-a-day running habit. See your doctor for a checkup and then build up slowly.

Fourth, learn to control stress. Hatha yoga, biofeedback, meditation, visualization techniques, breathing exercises, walking, and other methods will lower blood pressure. In one study, patients were hooked up to biofeedback instruments which let them know by the level of a sound how tense they were. Simultaneously the patients were taught to relax by paying attention to the process of breathing, by becoming consciously aware of every muscle, and by being certain that each muscle was relaxed. Mentally the patients repeated the word "relaxed" with every expiration. This entire program was practiced three times per week, one-half hour every time, for three months. Patients learned how to relax as evidenced by the biofeedback instruments. The result was a significant drop in both blood pressure and in the use of blood pressure-lowering drugs. The benefit lasted as long as the patients practiced the relaxation techniques.

So in the case of high blood pressure, as with many other diseases, the cause and solution are in the lifestyle. About 90% of all people with high blood pressure can solve their health problem in a safe and natural way.

« « « ◯ » » »

CANCER

Cancer is the scourge of the 20th century. The diagnosis of cancer is often like a death sentence. Even with all the advances in cancer research, over 50% of the people who develop cancer die within five years.

Remember when considering the subject of cancer that cancer is not just one disease but a multitude. Each type of cancer varies in type of treatment, length of time one might live, cause, and many other factors. Even though cancer of the breast and of the lung are both cancers, the differences are greater than the similarities.

When it comes to cancer, the most hopeful aspect is prevention. Once the condition has developed there are few viable solutions. Chemotherapy and surgery are distasteful, traumatic and usually ineffective. Laetrile, megavitamin therapy, herbs, DMSO, colonics, and other such approaches are of no proven value. Until scientific proof is presented, I recommend that people not waste time and resources in these directions.

What about prevention? Can we work to prevent cancer? Happily, the answer is yes. First, we should discuss some of the theories on how cancer is caused.

There are two main intriguing theories in scientific literature. The first is the oxygen starvation theory. Normal body cells require oxygen to live, yet most cancer cells do not need oxygen. Some studies have found that when normal cells are deprived of oxygen then these cells have two choices: die or convert to a type of cell which does not need oxygen. The cells choose the latter path, yet this conversion results in a more primitive form of cell which grows uncontrollably. In this way a cancer is formed. The most common cause of oxygen starvation is fat deposits in blood vessels.

The other theory of cancer development is the toxin concept. If normal cells are exposed repeatedly to irritating and toxic chemicals from a poor diet, the cells convert to a cancer form to

« « « ◯ » » »

survive.

There are many other theories of cancer development. Some scientists think that the body's system of resistance, the immune system, stops working properly and fails to destroy cancer cells as they develop in the normal course of life. Others believe that abnormal hormone levels will cause cancer cells to develop. There are almost as many theories as there are scientists. The bottom line is that no one knows for sure why cancer develops.

But scientists do know about measures that can be taken to prevent cancer from occurring. What can you do to protect yourself?

The first, and most obvious, is don't smoke. We all know that this is the number one step in cancer prevention.

Second, avoid a high fat diet. Eating large amounts of meat, dairy products, and eggs, besides increasing the risk of a heart attack, will raise the risk of cancer. Specifically, cancer of the breast, colon, skin, and prostate occur more frequently in people who eat too much fat.

To prevent heart disease, people have been advised to substitute unsaturated fats such as vegetable oils for the saturated fats found in animals foods. When this substitution is made, the risk of heart disease will decline, but the risk of cancer will increase. A diet high in unsaturated fats is therefore not healthful. Instead of substituting one form of fat for another it is best to reduce the total amount of fat in the diet.

The third measure which we can take to prevent cancer is to eat large amounts of fruits (especially citrus), vegetables, and whole grains (rice, bread, oats, etc.). The best vegetables are broccoli, cabbage, cauliflower, brussel sprouts, and carrots. There are protective factors against cancer found in these foods that have not been definitely identified. Taking vitamin and mineral tablets is no substitute.

Fourth, avoid overeating. Eating too much has been shown to be a major cause of cancer. In experiments, 100 rats, bred so that all develop cancer by the age of one year, were separated into two groups. One group was given all the standard rat chow they could eat, while the other group was given the same food but only in

« « « ◯ » » »

limited amounts. All rats in the first group, but only 20% of the rats in the restricted group developed cancer. This type of experiment has been performed at the finest cancer research institutes in the world many times.

Fifth, avoid foods containing nitrate, a chemical used to keep meat pink and to inhibit bacterial growth. Nitrate is found in preserved meats (bologna, hot dogs, salami, etc.), fish, and some cheeses. It has a proven connection with cancer.

Sixth, avoid saccharin, for it has been proven to cause cancer. If you are convinced that this is not true, it is because of a high-powered advertising campaign by the saccharin manufacturers to discredit the testing which showed that saccharin causes cancer. When saccharin was tested, doses were used that are far in excess of what the average person could consume. But only 100 rats were used to see if saccharin could cause one cancer in 10,000 people. Because 10,000 rats could not be used, the dose of saccharin was increased to compensate. This method is recognized as valid by all cancer researchers.

Sixth, do not broil or barbecue foods. This type of cooking results in the formation of benzopyrene, a powerful cancer-causing chemical, especially in sausage, fish, beef, steak, ribs, pork chops, and chicken.

Seventh, avoid foods containing food colorings. Many of these chemicals have been found to cause cancer and have been removed from foods. Public interest groups such as those formed by Ralph Nader are presently trying to get other colorings banned since they have been linked with cancer. Better to be safe than sorry: with a little effort, you can totally eliminate these chemicals from your diet.

Eighth, wash food carefully to eliminate as much of the insecticide residue as you can. Endrin, found on apples and wheat, has been linked to cancer.

Nine, minimize intake of salt-cured, salt-pickled, or smoked foods.

Ten, consume alcoholic beverages only in moderation or not at all.

Overall, close to 90% of all cancers are caused by lifestyle and

« « « ◯ » » »

environmental factors. Following the ten anti-cancer measures outlined above will decrease the chance of cancer by approximately 90%. Although the news about cancer treatment is often negative, the facts concerning cancer prevention are very positive. Doctors may not have great success in treating cancer, but you can probably avoid getting this disease in the first place by following a few simple suggestions. As always, an ounce of prevention is worth a pound of cure.

« « « ◯ » » »

DIABETES

Diabetes is a common ailment in the United States. It has been estimated that approximately 4.2 million people in our country have diabetes. Four out of every five diabetics are over 45 years old.

Most people believe that the cause of diabetes is unknown, the only successful treatment is drugs, and the common diabetes medications are effective and safe. Unfortunately, these are dangerous misconceptions.

Is the cause of diabetes unknown? No. In 85% of cases, the cause is clearly known to be overweight in combination with an inherited tendency for diabetes which would never be expressed if the person were of normal weight. When people who develop diabetes in adulthood lose enough weight, all evidence of diabetes disappears and no drug treatment is needed.

The only exception is with children who develop what is called juvenile diabetes, constituting about 15% of all cases of diabetes. Weight loss is usually not recommended since these diabetics are already thin. Medication is required. Occasionally a juvenile diabetic can be helped with dietary changes, but this is the exception.

In one study, a doctor followed the course of diabetes in an obese woman who lost weight and then gained the weight back months later. In the beginning when the woman weighed 209 pounds, her blood sugar and insulin levels were abnormally high as is found with severe diabetes. The woman then went on a strict diet and lost 80 pounds. Measurements of blood sugar and insulin levels showed that they were normal. Eight months later the woman again weighed 209 pounds as a result of extreme overeating. With this weight gain, the blood tests again showed evidence of severe diabetes.

Scientists consider this case typical of all cases of adult-onset diabetes. Clearly, then, the main cause of this condition is overweight. There is no mystery. But once the condition has

« « « ◯ » » »

developed what should a person do? Should drugs be used? Since almost all adult-onset diabetics can eliminate the illness with dietary changes, drugs are usually not necessary, but some people feel that the diet changes are more painful than taking drugs for a lifetime. Medications seem to be a safe and easy answer.

But this is not the case. All diabetes medications cause some degree of harm to the body. In fact, a study done in Poland found that the death rate of diabetics was highest in those treated with insulin (which must be injected), next highest in those treated with oral drugs, and lowest in those treated with diet alone.

When insulin was first developed it was regarded as a wonder drug. Although injected insulin will lower the blood sugar level it will also raise the risk of heart attacks, strokes, and high blood pressure. Apparently high levels of insulin increase the amount of fat deposited on the walls of blood vessels.

The oral diabetes drugs also increase the risk of heart disease and stroke. So we must conclude that there is a price to be paid for drug treatment.

Therefore it is clearly superior to control diabetes with diet instead of drugs. With dietary changes it is possible to eliminate almost all evidence of adult-onset diabetes.

For many years diabetics were told to eat less carbohydrates. This class of food includes starches and sugars. With digestion the starches are broken down into sugars. Diabetics have high blood levels of sugar, so it was thought that if they ate less of the foods that turn into sugar, they would reduce their blood sugar level.

But in the 1970s the experts changed their minds and concluded that they had been wrong. Studies began to show that a high carbohydrate diet was better for diabetics since it "turned on" the body systems needed for proper handling of sugar. Also, the low carbohydrate diets that had been used for years were found to increase greatly the risk of heart disease and strokes because they were so high in fats.

Further studies have shown that the best type of high carbohydrate diet is one that is also high in dietary fiber. Fiber is the part of food which cannot be digested and helps the body to maintain lower blood levels of sugar and fats. High fiber

« « « ○ » » »

carbohydrate foods are vegetables, fruits, grains, and cereals.

The Pritikin Center for diet and exercise recently published a study with 60 diabetics. The therapeutic diet consisted primarily of high fiber carbohydrates such as vegetables, grains and cereals. The diet was very low in fatty foods such as meats, dairy products, and eggs. Subjects were encouraged to walk daily and at the end of the study the average amount of time spent walking was almost two hours per day.

This program led to a dramatic improvement for almost all patients. Close to 90% of the diabetics who had been on drugs before initiating this diet and exercise program required no drugs at the end.

Therefore, the most modern scientific research has proven that the healthiest diabetic diet is one that uses very small amounts of high fat and refined low fiber carbohydrate foods. It is easy to get fat by eating these foods since they supply many calories relative to how full you feel after eating them. One candy bar contains 250 calories but it will not fill you up as much as if you eat three apples supplying the same number of calories. High fat and refined carbohydrate foods also interfere with the body's effort to maintain normal blood sugar levels and they elevate blood fat levels.

The high fat foods are meats, dairy products, eggs, oil, nuts and seeds. Refined carbohydrates foods are cookies, candy, cake, soda pop, white bread, white rice, donuts, etc.

The foods to eat a lot of are vegetables, fruits, and whole grains (whole wheat bread, brown rice, etc.). The quantity of food must be kept low enough that normal weight is maintained. Exercise will help with this goal.

Adult-onset diabetes is an excellent example of the fact that most major diseases can be controlled by lifestyle changes. Diabetics can choose between a healthy life or one punctuated by blindness, heart attacks, amputations, and other serious problems. We cannot rely upon drugs to prevent these complications. But a healthful diet can change adult-onset diabetes from a dangerous life-threatening disease to simply a bad memory.

« « « 〇 » » »

HYPOGLYCEMIA

Are you tired all the time? If so, chances are that someone has told you that you may have hypoglycemia. That "someone" was probably a well-meaning friend, but it could have been a doctor.

What is hypoglycemia? It is low blood sugar. Typical symptoms which occur when the blood sugar level drops below normal are sweating, shaking, fast heartbeat, nervousness, weakness, fatigue, hunger, nausea, headaches, restlessness, and unclear thinking.

I am sure that halfway through this list many readers have begun to suspect that they have hypoglycemia. But most people will occasionally have headaches, fatigue, restlessness, and other typical symptoms of hypoglycemia even if they do not really have this disease. The list of conditions which will cause these symptoms includes anemia, heart disease, brain tumors, the flu, and many other common illnesses.

How can you know for sure if you have hypoglycemia? Because you cannot depend on the symptoms, other methods must be used. The standard test for hypoglycemia is the glucose tolerance test. With this test a person will fast for 10 hours and then have his blood sugar level checked. Next a large dose of sugar is swallowed in the form of syrup. One-half hour later the blood sugar level is again tested. Following this the blood sugar level is checked every hour for five to six hours.

After fasting ten hours the blood sugar is expected to be normal. When the sugar is ingested the blood sugar will rise rapidly. After a few hours the level should return to normal. If the sugar level drops way below normal before returning to the normal level, hypoglycemia may be present.

This test is used almost universally but there are some major problems with it. One is that the patient is usually not asked how he felt during the course of the test. If he felt perfectly fine when his blood sugar dropped below normal, then we cannot say that his hypoglycemic-like symptoms are from hypoglycemia. We can

« « « ◯ » » »

only be sure that the symptoms are from hypoglycemia if they occur when the blood sugar level is low.

The other major problem is that the glucose tolerance test is performed in an artificial situation. Very few people would fast for 10 hours and then drink a large quantity of overwhelmingly sweet syrup. It might even be safe to say that it would be normal for people to get sick from this type of experience.

Many people erroneously consider themselves to be hypoglycemic based on symptoms alone. Others make the error of depending upon the unreliable glucose tolerance test. Fortunately however, there is a very simple way to definitely determine if hypoglycemia exists.

If you suspect hypoglycemia have your doctor give you a written prescription for a blood sugar test. With this test you only need to have blood checked one time, you do not need to fast, and you don't have to drink sugar syrup. Keep the prescription handy and when you feel the symptoms that you think may be related to hypoglycemia, immediately go to the laboratory and have your blood sugar level checked. If your sugar level is normal *at the exact time* that you're feeling weak, shaky, tired, etc., then your symptoms are not from hypoglycemia. If your sugar level is below normal, then you have hypoglycemia.

When hypoglycemia is tested for in this way it is very rare to find that the symptoms are from low blood sugar. For every one case of true hypoglycemia there are probably 100 people who blame their symptoms on hypoglycemia when there is another cause altogether. Most people who suspect that they have hypoglycemia in fact are suffering from toxemia (see chapter on this subject).

But let's say that we actually have found someone with hypoglycemia. The next step is to determine which type since this will determine what course of action the person will need to follow to solve his problem.

There are two main types of hypoglycemia. The first type is called fasting hypoglycemia since it occurs when a person has gone many hours without food. The second type is called non-fasting or reactive hypoglycemia since it occurs after a person has

« « « ◯ » » »

eaten the wrong food and it is a reaction to this food.

Fasting hypoglycemia is very rare and serious. People with this type of hypoglycemia are usually extremely ill and in need of hospitalization due to the underlying condition which is causing the low blood sugar. The typical causes of fasting hypoglycemia include excessive intake of drugs used by diabetics to lower the blood sugar level; serious adrenal gland, liver, or kidney problems; chronic alcoholism; and tumors in the pancreas gland.

Non-fasting hypoglycemia is slightly less rare than the fasting type. It usually results from eating too much sugar. Because sugar requires very little time to be digested, it easily rushes from the intestines into the bloodstream. The blood sugar level will then shoot up and in response the pancreas gland will secrete a large amount of insulin to lower the blood sugar level. Sometimes too much insulin is secreted and the blood sugar level is knocked down too far. When the sugar level drops way below normal the common symptoms of hypoglycemia occur.

Hypoglycemia of any type is extremely rare. But if it is found that you have hypoglycemia, what should you do? The standard remedy is proper diet and the typical diet used is one high in protein. A high protein diet is used because protein is converted very slowly into blood sugar and therefore it will not rapidly elevate the sugar level as will regular white sugar. No excessive secretion of insulin will result so the blood sugar level will not drop below normal.

But even though a high protein diet will help stabilize the blood sugar level, it will also cause many serious health problems. The list of such problems includes acceleration of the aging process, increased buildup of fat in the blood vessels (which is the cause of heart attacks and strokes), and the brittle bone condition called osteoporosis (see chapter on protein). Fortunately there is an alternative to the high-protein diet which will solve the problem of hypoglycemia without developing other health problems.

The best diet for hypoglycemia is one high in complex carbohydrates such as vegetables, grains and cereals (brown rice, whole wheat bread, etc.) Therefore the sugar which is formed

« « « ◯ » » »

when these foods are digested will slowly trickle into the bloodstream, as opposed to the rush of sugar which results from eating simple carbohydrates. A diet high in complex carbohydrates will solve the problem of hypoglycemia without causing any new health problems as will the high-protein diet.

The "bad" carbohydrates, the ones which will cause hypoglycemia and should be avoided, are sugar, honey, cake, candy, soda pop, and all other super-sweet foods. The best results come from a diet which is high in vegetables, moderate in grains and fruits, and low in high fat foods (meats, dairy products, eggs, nuts, seeds, etc.).

As fruit is sweet, should it also be avoided? No. Since the sugar in an unprocessed piece of fruit is attached to fiber, it is absorbed into the bloodstream slowly. Because of this, fruits do not usually cause hypoglycemia. When fruit is juiced, however, the fruit sugar is released from the fiber. Juices can cause almost as much trouble as white sugar and they therefore should be avoided.

There is scientific evidence that alcoholic and caffeinated beverages can cause hypoglycemia. The martini taken for relaxation and the coffee used to produce a "lift" in energy, may knock the blood sugar level down low enough to cause hypoglycemic symptoms. Therefore it is best to avoid these beverages.

Hypoglycemia is a rare but troublesome condition. Don't assume that you have it just because your symptoms are typical of hypoglycemia. And don't rely on the glucose tolerance test. Ask your doctor to use the simple test outlined above. And, if you have hypoglycemia, follow a diet high in complex carbohydrates such as the one described in this book, rather than one high in protein. You will find that hypoglycemia is easy to diagnose accurately and easy to eliminate through healthful living.

« « « ◯ » » »

SLOWING THE AGING PROCESS

For centuries people have been looking for ways to live longer. They have tried medicines, elixirs, special foods and waters, megavitamins and other products of the laboratory. Countless other potential answers to aging have been experimented with for centuries.

To the disappointment of many, these supposed anti-aging potions do not work, and many are harmful. Gerontologists (experts in aging) have investigated anti-aging potions and foods in depth and have found them all to be worthless.

There is a way, however, that you can prolong your lifespan by *CHANGING YOUR DIET.* Scientific evidence shows that you can live longer by eating less food.

Scholars of the Bible and of general history do not find this surprising. In 3800 B.C. the following inscription was made in an Egyptian pyramid: "Man lives on one fourth of what he eats. On the other three fourths lives his doctor." In the Bible, Ecclesiastes 37:31 says: "Many have died of gluttony, but he who is careful to avoid it prolongs his life." Temperance in eating and drinking to prolong life also was discussed in the early Chinese writing of Huang Ti.

In the 20th century hundreds of scientists have studied the effect of food restriction on aging. The first large scale research was done in the 1930s by a doctor at Cornell University. Dozens of experiments showed that when one group of animals was fed an adequate diet in restricted amounts while another group of animals was allowed to eat all they wanted of the same food, the restricted group lived 50% longer. Lifespan was prolonged because there was lower incidence of chronic diseases.

Since the 1930s the research at Cornell has been confirmed many times in all forms of life from protozoa to fish to rats. The

« « « O » » »

general conclusion is that if the amount of calories is restricted so that no excess fat accumulates, the length of life will be significantly prolonged.

But what about the effect of diet in humans? Obviously scientists cannot study people directly by locking them in laboratories and juggling their diets for a lifetime. However insurance company statistics indirectly support the research work done with non-human forms of life. Such statistics show that overweight people have higher risks of heart disease, strokes, kidney and liver diseases, appendicitis, problems in pregnancy and childbirth, hernia, degenerative joint diseases, cancer, and lung diseases.

The scientific community has concluded, therefore, that overeating in both animals and human beings will increase the risk of many diseases and shorten the lifespan. It is a fact that "the longer the belt line, the shorter the life line."

There are five main theories which explain the nature of the aging process. Eating less food has been proven with each theory to prolong lifespan.

The cross-linkage theory of aging explains the wrinkling of the skin and stiffening of the joints which occurs later in life. With aging, increased numbers of fibers (cross-links) form between particles of connective tissue (collagen). This causes a loss of elasticity and makes the tissue more brittle. Studies have shown that the process of cross-linkage can be retarded by restricting food intake.

The endocrine gland theory of aging states that aging is a normal process that may be speeded up by increased thyroid gland activity. Such an increase would make the organs work harder and therefore age faster. Eating less food decreases thyroid gland activity.

The growth rate theory of aging holds that the body which grows at the fastest rate will live the shortest amount of time. Experiments have shown that overeating speeds up the growth rate while eating the amount of food which the body actually needs will slow the growth rate and prolong the lifespan.

The genetic code error theory proposes that the more the

« « « ◯ » » »

cellular genetic code of DNA and RNA is used, the sooner it will show age-related imperfections. The genetic code is the inner "computer program" of the cell which determines the type of work to be done by each cell. Eating less food, and especially avoiding an overdose of protein, will reduce the use of this code, thus delaying the onset of age-related imperfections.

The last major theory of aging addresses the accumulation of waste products inside the cells. It is thought that such substances are harmful enough to speed up the aging process. Eating too much food will increase the amount of waste products inside cells.

The conclusion is that eating the proper amount of food and avoiding overeating will prolong the lifespan for many reasons that can be theoretically explained and understood.

The best time to start an anti-aging dietary program is at birth. Breast-feeding will help since it provides for slower growth when compared to other types of feeding and this will prolong the lifespan. It is best to feed an infant with nothing besides breast milk for the first four to six months of life.

In adult life there are many ways to cut down on the amount of calories without feeling hungry all the time. Strive to fill up on low calories foods at the expense of high calorie foods. This means eating mainly vegetables and fruits. One pound of celery contains 58 calories; one pound of apples, 242 calories; one pound of whole wheat bread, 1100 calories; one pound of cheese, 1840 calories; one pound of steak, 1760 calories.

The high calorie foods are almost always high in fat. The list of high fat foods includes oil, shortening, butter, margarine, bacon, salad dressings, meats, poultry, fish, dairy products, nuts, and eggs. A diet plan can only be low in calories if very minimal amounts of high fat foods are eaten.

Studies have shown that an intake of vitamins higher than the recommended dietary allowance (RDA) will prolong the lifespan. The diet described in this book supplies such a higher level of vitamins. Eating one and a half carrots and two oranges per day would provide three times the RDA of vitamin C and 1.7 times that of vitamin A. Also, the diet is rich in vitamin E (the best foods

« « « ◯ » » »

for E are dark green leafy vegetables, nuts and legumes) and low in polyunsaturated fatty acids which increase the need for E.

As with most aspects of health, diet is not everything. Exercising vigorously (aerobically) four or five times per week will help keep body weight at a minimum and will have many other anti-aging effects.

You can live longer, enjoy more health, and have more energy simply by making easy changes in the way you live. The true "Fountain of Youth" is within your reach.

« « « O » » »

OSTEOPOROSIS

Osteoporosis is a serious problem which occurs primarily in women. After menopause, when the level of estrogen secretion falls, women lose bone at a fast rate. As the bone becomes more porous and brittle, it becomes much easier to break. A brush up against a table or a fall to the ground may fracture a bone. What can be done to prevent osteoporosis or reverse it once it is present?

Many people believe that osteoporosis is caused by a dietary deficiency of calcium and that a cure can be produced by taking large amounts of calcium. But the truth is not so simple. Osteoporosis is not a calcium deficiency disease and calcium supplements have not been proven to strengthen bone.

In fact, osteoporosis is not primarily from loss of bone calcium, but rather from loss of the fibers in bone upon which calcium is deposited.

Nonetheless, some studies have shown benefit from maintaining adequate amounts of calcium in the body. But ingesting large amounts of calcium may not be the best way to assure optimal body calcium levels.

A dietary calcium deficiency is often cited as the cause of osteoporosis because statistics show that most Americans do not consume the Recommended Dietary Allowance (RDA) or 800 milligrams (mgs) of calcium per day. But the story does not end here. The 1980 edition of Recommended Dietary Allowances also says that "adults remain in calcium balance despite lower calcium intakes." The World Health Organization is quoted as saying that "a practical allowance for adults should be between 400 and 500 mgs per day because there appeared to be no evidence of calcium deficiency in countries in which calcium intakes were of this order." The observation is made that: "Studies have shown that men adapt with time to lower calcium intakes and maintain calcium balance on intakes as low as 200—400 mgs per day."

Why, if a less than 800 mgs of calcium per day is totally

« « « ◯ » » »

adequate, does the National Research Council recommend 800 milligrams? Because of the "high levels of protein and phosphorus provided by the United States diet." Studies have found that "calcium losses can be substantial when protein intake is high" and "high phosphate intakes... enhance bone loss in mice and rats."

The RDA text clearly states that people who consume less than the usual amount of protein and phosphorus will be safe with a calcium intake "considerably" lower than 800 mg. per day. Meats and dairy products are the primary sources of both protein and phosphorus, so if we do not overdose on these foods we will not develop a calcium deficiency if less than 800 mgs per day are consumed.

A considerable amount of scientific research proves that meat and dairy products are the primary causes of heart disease, many types of cancer, strokes, and other health problems. To prevent these illnesses, it is best to either greatly reduce or eliminate the use of meat and dairy foods. When we decrease our intake of these foods, then the need for calcium will be reduced to the point where 400–500 mgs. per day will be more than enough.

It is ironic that the food most often promoted as preventing osteoporosis, namely milk, is a potential cause of osteoporosis because of its high content of protein and phosphorus.

Treating osteoporosis with calcium supplements has never been consistently proven to be helpful. In one recent study, 103 post-menopausal women filled out diet questionnaires and were divided into three groups based on calcium intake: those with an intake below 550 mg. per day, those with an intake between 550 mg. and 1150 mg. per day, and those with an intake above 1150 mg. per day. All of the women were given supplements of 500 mg. calcium per day to be used in addition to their normal dietary intake. After two years, all three groups showed a similar worsening of osteoporosis.

In another study, a group of fourteen women with osteoporosis were given a 1000 mg. supplement of calcium daily for eight days. Changes in chemicals excreted in the urine seemed to

« « « ◯ » » »

indicate a slowing of the osteoporotic process.

Today most experts believe that a high calcium intake will not help, prevent, or reverse osteoporosis. Still, it is prudent to be sure that we have enough calcium stored in the body.

There are two ways to increase the amount of calcium in the body. The first is to ingest more calcium in the form of food or supplements. The second is to eat less protein which will result in less calcium being lost in the urine. Consider the pros and cons of these two methods.

Excessive calcium intake may increase the chance of kidney stones and decrease the absorption of manganese and zinc, two important minerals. Therefore it is best to avoid taking excessive amounts of calcium if there is an alternative way to assure adequate calcium supplies in the body.

A high protein intake will increase the risk of heart disease and strokes, accelerate the aging process, and cause more calcium to be eliminated from the body (see chapter on protein). Therefore it is best to avoid a high protein intake.

Because both excessive calcium and high protein intake cause many health problems, it is best to avoid overdoses of both nutrients. If a low but safe amount of protein is ingested, the calcium requirement will be so low that a proper diet will supply sufficient calcium to maintain optimal levels in the body. This is the most rational and healthful course to follow.

Estrogen is often prescribed to help prevent osteoporosis. But estrogen has side effects that are more dangerous than osteoporosis. The list of the side effects of estrogen includes uterine cancer, gall bladder disease, blood clots (which may cause a heart attack), liver tumors, elevated blood pressure, and worsening of diabetes.

If you do not have osteoporosis, you can do quite a bit to prevent it. We have already discussed the healthful anti-osteoporosis diet which is low in protein. This diet is high in foods such as vegetables, grains, nuts, and seeds which contain the necessary amounts of calcium. But another major factor is exercise.

Exercise has been proven to strengthen bone in the same way

« « « ◯ » » »

that it strengthens muscle. For instance, it is commonly found that a right-handed tennis player will have larger muscles in his right arm. One study of such tennis players found that the bone in the right arm will also be larger from the extra activity. The rule "use it or lose it" applies here. The bones of the body require regular exercise to maintain their strength and density. This does not mean you need to run ten miles a day. A brisk walk of one mile per day and using the upper body to do yard and house work will probably do the job.

Sufficient vitamin D is needed so that the intestines will absorb the calcium we eat. With moderate exposure of the skin to the sun the body will produce plenty of this vitamin.

Once osteoporosis has developed there are no proven remedies. But if we eat properly and exercise regularly, we can either prevent or slow the progress of this condition. (See the chapter on calcium and dairy products for more information relevant to a discussion of osteoporosis.)

« « « ◯ » » »

ALLERGIES
& ASTHMA

Spring comes, the air warms, flowers bloom, trees leaf out, and many people wheeze and sneeze so much that they long for winter. Is there hope for allergy sufferers or must they spend months with tissue paper and antihistamines at hand?

Allergies and asthma are considered by many to be purely the body's reaction to inhalation or ingestion of irritating substances. Pollen, house dust, cat hair, dairy products, eggs: these are all common examples of noxious substances.

But as is true with infections (see chapter on infectious diseases), one cannot look at the irritating substances in a vacuum. They must be considered relative to the health and resistance of the body. A healthy body is better able to deal with environmental irritants such as dust and pollen.

Food allergies are another subject altogether. Most foods to which people are allergic are abnormal foods in a human diet. Cow's milk products are the most common food to which people are allergic. But cow's milk is specifically designed for baby cows, not baby human beings. There are vast chemical differences between cow's milk and human milk. Cow's milk clearly is not a normal food for human beings, so if people become ill after eating cheese or drinking milk there should be no surprise.

The most common foods to which people are allergic are cow's milk products, wheat and other cereals, eggs, chicken, beef, fish, and citrus. There are many tests for food allergies including skin and blood tests. But the most reliable approach is an elimination diet which uses the body as the laboratory.

Most of the foods to which people are allergic can be found in the typical daily menu. Therefore most people will have some amount of the irritating food inside the body at all times. Since the food provokes allergy symptoms, some degree of symptoms will

« « « O » » »

be present at all times. Typical symptoms include abdominal pain, vomiting, diarrhea, asthma, runny nose, and skin rashes.

With an elimination diet all of the common allergy-producing foods are avoided for one to two weeks. During this period of time most allergy-related symptoms will disappear. After the symptoms have subsided, foods are introduced one at a time. For two days the relatively safe foods which have been eaten on the elimination diet will be eaten with milk. Then, for the next two days, milk is omitted and wheat is substituted. Each suspected food is tested in this way. When the person eats a food to which he is allergic, the symptoms will be very clear since there has been a complete absence of symptoms for the past week or two on the elimination diet. In this way, a diet can be created which is free of all foods to which the patient is allergic.

Allergies to environmental substances such as pollen and dust are common. In contrast to food allergies, it is not abnormal for human beings to be exposed to such chemicals. Therefore the approach with environmental allergens is to strengthen the body so much that it is not troubled when exposed.

People who become extremely ill during pollen season invariably are on a poor diet with insufficient exercise and rest plus an overdose of stress. They resemble a forest after a long drought: one tiny spark will produce a catastrophe. But after a few months of sensible eating, sufficient physical activity, plenty of rest, and a reduction in stress, the person will become more like a drenched forest: lighter fluid and matches could not start a fire.

It is rare for someone to become totally free of allergic symptoms. But when progress has been made to the extent that a person sneezes once or twice when mowing the lawn instead of becoming paralyzed with asthma, both doctor and patient will be satisfied. This is the common outcome of a health improvement program with allergic people.

Asthma is considered an allergic-type illness. People who eat a food that is inappropriate for human consumption, or who inhale irritating pollens in conjunction with a weakened system, are thrown into a crisis. The muscles around the bronchial tubes (the pipes that carry air from the throat to the lungs) tighten up so

« « « ◯ » » »

much that air cannot get into or out of the lungs. The person feels like he is suffocating. Emergency rooms are very familiar with asthma because people sometimes come for treatment to save their lives.

The drugs used with asthma range from theophylline and marax to cortisone. Most doctors feel that there is no alternative to drugs for asthmatics. Yet this is far from the truth. The same measures that work with other allergy sufferers also work with asthmatics. If one eats rationally and learns to relax, asthma will usually disappear. Depending on the case, this may be easy or difficult to achieve. But under the direction of an experienced doctor, good results are almost always achieved. Rare failures are usually linked to years of cortisone use. This drug, often called the king of all drugs, is also the king killer of all drugs. As miraculous as the short term results of cortisone use may seem to be, the long term results are equally disastrous. Problems commonly seen are destruction of bone, muscle, skin, glands, and many other tissues. The body's healing power is weakened so much that a health-building program will have much less impact. The morale: avoid cortisone as much as humanly possible.

In 1980, I worked with a man suffering from severe asthma. The results were so dramatic that I wish to share the details with you.

The man, Jim Worster (not his actual name), was 65 years old and retired from his work as a PhD. college professor. He had been suffering from severe asthma for over seven years. His symptoms were a continuous loud wheeze on breathing, a frequent harsh barking cough, and a gurgling sound in his lungs from fluid buildup. It was so difficult for Jim to breath that he was exhausted most of the time. Previous treatment consisted of aminophylline for seven years and marax for one year.

The patient came in on September 14, 1980. For the first two weeks, he ate exclusively raw vegetable salads and oranges. At the end of this period of time, his symptoms were much less severe. During the next two weeks, Jim fasted, drinking only distilled water. Two days after beginning the fast, all of Jim's asthma symptoms disappeared and he stopped taking all drugs. The fast

« « « ○ » » »

was ended on October 12, and then Jim ate only fruits and vegetables for two more weeks. At the end of this period, Jim was discharged free of any symptoms of asthma, needing no drugs, and 11 pounds lighter.

On November 26 I received a letter from Jim. In it he stated: "I think I may say that my session (of dieting and fasting) was one of the most exciting experiences of my life, and it was doubly gratifying to experience such relief of my asthmatic condition. My thanks to all of you."

Another case which illustrates the effectiveness of proper diet is a little boy who we will call Bill. His parents brought him in at the age of ten months. Bill had suffered from chronic severe middle ear infections for four months, had taken antibiotics every day, and now was being considered for surgical placement of tubes in the ears to improve drainage.

To resolve this problem Bill was fed only fruits and vegetables for two weeks. After one week, his parents took him off of the antibiotics. When the two week period ended, Bill was completely well. He had no fever, no ear infections, and no chronic fatigue as before. His diet was broadened to include grains, cereals, and small amounts of chicken and fish but no dairy products. Two years have now passed and Bill has doubled in size and experienced no further ear infections or health problems of any type.

With allergies and asthma the message is the same as with most health disturbances: improve your health by living more healthfully and you will say goodbye to most or all of your problems. The majority of allergy and asthma sufferers will be able to give up their medications and feel great.

« « « ◯ » » »

INFECTIOUS DISEASES

What is the cause of infectious diseases? With such illnesses, the body has apparently been invaded by dangerous bacteria and viruses. Most people have been taught that bacteria and viruses are the sole cause of infections. Is this the truth?

No. The top medical pathology textbook, by Robbins, states that: "Bacterial disease-producing potential is relative to the resistance of the host (the human body). Man lives in a relatively delicate state of balance with his microbial environment. He is in constant contact with a wide range of bacteria, viruses, fungi, and indeed, all manner of microbiologic agents with whom he lives in a state of commensalism (mutual cooperation)." The author further says that bacteria and viruses are present on all body surfaces and in every body opening (ears, nose, throat, etc.) at all times and that, under normal conditions, these organisms are harmless.

Harrison's *Principles of Internal Medicine* states that the mere presence of an infection-causing organism in the body does not "lead invariably to clinical illness. Indeed, the production of symptoms in man by many parasites (such as viruses and bacteria) is the exception rather than the rule, and the subclinical infection or the 'carrier state' is the usual host-parasite relationship." The terms "subclinical infection" and "carrier state" mean that the bacteria or virus is living in the body but causing no illness whatsoever.

Harrison further states that "even rabies virus infection, which was at one time believed to nearly always cause progressive fatal disease in nearly all instances, has been shown to produce a significant number of subclinical infections in both animals and man." Rabies virus traditionally has been considered one of the most dangerous of all organisms. Yet even this virus can

« « « ◯ » » »

be found living in perfectly healthy men and animals and be incapable of causing disease.

The list of bacteria and fungi which can be found living on a healthy body includes streptococci, the alleged cause of "strep" throat, and candida, the alleged cause of many serious yeast infections. Since such dangerous organisms can be found living in healthy bodies, how can anyone claim that they are the sole cause of disease?

The only logical conclusion is that bacteria and viruses are not the sole cause of infection. An infection will not develop unless the body's resistance to infection is lowered due to poor health. Instead of waging war on bacteria and viruses, we should try to increase resistance.

To do this, one must improve health, and health can only be improved by living more healthfully. Healthful living consists of eating the right foods in proper amounts, exercising regularly, avoiding excessive stress, getting plenty of rest, breathing unpolluted air, and drinking pure water. If a person were to follow these practices exactly as required, he would gain almost complete immunity to infectious diseases.

Science has clearly shown that malnutrition will lower resistance. Deficiences of protein and/or vitamins will lead to infections. Such deficiences are almost never found in the United States, but in the third world countries.

There is a form of malnutrition that is epidemic in our country: overnutrition. Scientific and historical studies have proven that overeating can cause infection.

In the 1830s in England, jails had to tell the government every year exactly how much they had spent on each prisoner for food. It was found that the more food consumed, the greater likelihood of infection. In a World War II concentration camp, almost 100% of the "well-fed" German guards died of typhus while only 30% of "mal-nourished" Russian prisoners died. Resistance was higher in the prisoners since they ate less food, but not so little an amount as to cause protein or vitamin deficiencies.

In a laboratory experiment, mice were infected with bacteria and then divided into two groups. One group was allowed to

« « « ◯ » » »

follow its inner instinct and not eat, but the second group was force-fed. The result was an increased death rate and shorter survival time in the mice that had eaten.

There are many possible reasons why overeating increases the chance of infection. When excess food is eaten, there is a buildup of excess food material inside the blood vessels, and inside and surrounding every one of the millions of cells in the body. When this material accumulates in too great an amount, the cells of the body will not be able to work properly, resistance to infection will be lowered and bacteria and viruses will be more able to thrive.

Another possible reason is explained by the "garbage can" analogy. When a garbage can is full, flies will swarm and maggots will proliferate. If the garbage can is empty and clean, flies will not propagate. When people overeat, there is a buildup of waste products which attract bacteria and viruses. If the body is not overloaded with food, it will efficiently remove waste products and the attraction for microorganisms will disappear. Bacteria and viruses may be nature's scavengers which aid the body in removing excess waste material.

Whatever the reason, it is known that overeating will increase the chance of infection. But diet is not everything. Stress, in the form of divorce, marriage, loss of job, change to a different job, change in residence, etc., also can increase the chance of infection. During a period of stress, the adrenal glands secrete more of certain hormones which suppress the functioning of the body's defensive systems, thus allowing unchecked bacterial and viral growth. One study found that with excessive stress, people are four times more likely to have a respiratory infection than if no serious emotional shock had been experienced.

Lack of rest is also a factor to consider. When the body gets too little rest, all of its functions are compromised. The elimination systems (liver, kidneys, etc.), are not able to do their full job of removing body waste products. Such materials will then accumulate excessively, and this may help cause an infection as mentioned previously. Also, lack of rest robs the body of the energy it needs to destroy bacteria and viruses.

« « « ◯ » » »

What course should be taken if an infection develops? Resort to drugs only if the infection is severe, such as pneumonia or kidney infection. If the infection is not this severe, such as is found with the common cold or the flu, it is best to avoid drugs. With an infection the body will initiate a major effort to heal itself and it is best if we cooperate.

With an infection appetite is lost. The body knows that eating when sick will divert energy from healing to digestion; therefore the brain turns off the appetite. Studies have shown that fasting during the course of an infection will increase the bacteria-killing ability of the body's defensive white blood cells. Furthermore, fasting allows the body to burn and/or eliminate some of the excess material which has accumulated in and around the cells. It is best to fast under professional supervision.

Fever is also found with infection. In the past, fever has been regarded as an enemy which should be suppressed. But scientists now recognize that fever is a beneficial part of the healing process. Studies have shown that bacteria and viruses are much more easily destroyed when the body temperature is raised. The brain may also turn up the intensity of the internal fires to burn up excessive waste material more rapidly. Therefore do not attempt to lower the fever with drugs unless it goes above 104 degrees, an extremely rare occurrence. Again, professional supervision is recommended.

Vomiting, diarrhea, sneezing, and coughing should all be regarded as defensive, healing activities initiated by the body to cleanse the system of waste products and allow healing to occur. As such they should not be suppressed by drugs except in those rare instances where they become a danger in and of themselves. This occurs approximately 5% of the time. In all other cases, vomiting will cease when the stomach is cleansed, diarrhea will stop when the intestines have become free of irritating wastes, sneezing will halt when the nasal passages are sufficiently drained of mucous, and coughing will end when the lungs have finished eliminating the wastes which had been choking these precious organs.

There is no denying that certain bacteria, such as those

« « « ⃝ » » »

involved with cholera and syphilis, are so strong that not even the healthiest person could resist invasion. Antibiotics may save lives in these cases. But with other infections, constituting 99% of cases in our country, the main cause is lowered resistance due to poor health. Rather than attacking bacteria and viruses, we should concentrate on building health.

ARTHRITIS

Aches and pains in joints are extremely common in middle and old age. In fact it is rare to see someone over the age of 45 who does not have some evidence of arthritis.

There are two major types of arthritis. The first, and most common, is osteoarthritis, also called degenerative joint disease, arthrosis, and spondylosis. The second major type of arthritis is called rheumatoid arthritis. It is far less common than osteoarthritis but it is usually far more serious.

How can you help yourself if you are suffering from one of these types of arthritis? Fortunately there are many lifestyle changes which will help. This is fortunate since most common anti-arthritis medications have serious side effects. Also, the drugs do not heal the arthritis. They simply reduce the severity of the symptoms while the underlying disease progresses.

What are some of the common arthritis drugs? Motrin is one, and its list of side effects includes nausea, heartburn, stomach ulcer, headache, skin rash, ringing in the ears, anemia, fluid retention, and others. Indocin is another, and its side effects are the same as with Motrin except for the headaches which are more frequent and more severe. Butazolidin is a third common anti-arthritis drug with most of the same side effects as the others. But it is unique in that it is the only arthritis drug in use today that consumer groups have petitioned the FDA to ban because of its toxicity.

Obviously, if at all possible, it is preferable to avoid arthritis drugs because of their many hazards.

Is there a safer alternative for arthritis? Is there a way to heal the joint inflammation which causes pain? In many cases the answer is yes. Dietary changes often have a dramatic effect.

The relation between rheumatoid arthritis and diet has been scientifically investigated with positive results. A case study from a London medical school showed that milk and cheese can aggravate this condition. Another study from Wayne State

« « « ◯ » » »

University found that six patients with rheumatoid arthritis became completely symptom-free when placed on a fat-free diet. Experiments with forty-four rheumatoid arthritis patients found that relief of pain and swelling resulted when certain foods were avoided, most commonly wheat, corn, and beef. A diet providing a relatively small amount of tryptophan, an amino acid subunit of protein, has been shown to relieve the pain of rheumatoid arthritis. These and many other studies have shown a link between rheumatoid arthritis and food.

Besides specific foods, the overall amount of food has been found to have an effect on rheumatoid arthritis. Total fasting has been proven to relieve the pain of this condition and result in positive changes in blood tests. Scientists have long known that a restricted food intake will reduce the severity of rheumatoid arthritis in animals.

The second major type of arthritis is osteoarthritis. At the Fourth International Food Allergy Symposium in July of 1982, Dr. Derek Wraith of the Memorial Hospital in London stated that "joint pain and swelling, the classic symptoms of arthritis, may actually be caused by food allergy in some patients." He successfully treated forty-two arthritis patients in England by removing eggs, milk, sugar, wheat, and yeast from their diets.

In support of Dr. Wraith's work, scientists have found that eating minimal amounts of food will slow the development of osteoarthritis in animals.

An example of the link between diet and arthritis is a patient with rheumatoid arthritis whom I worked with in 1980. We will call him Don Smith (not his real name). His first symptoms were shoulder pain in 1971 after overworking this joint. This pain lasted so long and became so severe that Don went to see a doctor. The initial diagnosis was tendinitis. Aspirin was prescribed but it was ineffective.

Suddenly the pain began to travel from joint to joint, affecting both shoulders, hands, feet, and knees. The M.D. next tried Butazolidin. When it was obvious that this drug was ineffective, Prednisone (a form of cortisone) was tried.

In 1972 this patient was sent to a rheumatologist who

« « « ◯ » » »

diagnosed rheumatoid arthritis. More drugs were prescribed including Plaquenil, Tandearil, Methotrexate, and an anti-depressant. Again there was little or no improvement.

In the next few years this patient went from doctor to doctor, trying different drug regimens including gold injections, Motrin, and sixteen aspirin per day. The drugs would help for a few months, then the pain would return. Drug side effects caused an abnormally low white blood cell count, imbalance in electrolytes, ringing in the ears, and many other problems.

Finally in 1980 after nine years of frustration, continued pain, and treatment with almost every conceivable arthritis drug, Don decided to try something different: a special diet and fasting. Initially Don's diet consisted of raw fruits and vegetables for nine days. During this period of time he slowly reduced his intake of aspirin and Prednisone so that, by the tenth day, he was on no medication whatsoever.

For the next three days, he ate a piece of fruit for breakfast and green juice (spinach, parsley, celery) for lunch and dinner. On the thirteenth day he started a total fast, ingesting only water.

During the first four days after stopping the medication, Don had pain all over his body and he was not able to sleep. On the fifth day, however, the pain dramatically reduced in severity. Don went on to fast a total of thirty-four days, with two periods of two days each during which he drank fruit and vegetable juices. The fast was ended with five days of fruit and vegetable juices, then thirteen days of raw fruits, raw and cooked vegetables, with the addition of rice the last five days.

At the end of his diet and fasting program, Don was experiencing only traces of pain even though he was on no medication. Three months later more severe pain had not returned and Don was planning another fast to get rid of the last traces of pain.

Rheumatoid arthritis is a very serious illness and to resolve it requires a firm commitment to a program of diet and fasting. But the benefits of such a program can be many years of life almost completely free of pain, plus freedom from medications and their side effects.

« « « ◯ » » »

Osteoarthritis is usually much easier to help than rheumatoid arthritis. A typical case of osteoarthritis is a 43 year old woman whom we will call Susan Jacobs (not her real name). Susan was suffering from severe osteoarthritic pain in her neck, upper back, and fingers. Her fingers were so stiff and painful that she could barely type; this threatened her livelihood as a secretary.

Susan was initially put on a two week diet program consisting exclusively of raw fruits and vegetables. At the end of the two weeks Susan was able to bend her fingers as far as is normal without pain. Also, the pain in her neck and upper back was greatly reduced. Susan's case is typical of what most osteoarthritics will experience following this type of dietary change.

To help either rheumatoid arthritis or osteoarthritis, it is initially necessary to follow a very strict diet and/or fasting. After the condition has improved, a more liberal diet may be used such as those described in the back of this book.

Remember that arthritis is an inflammation of the joints. Inflammation, as discussed in a previous chapter, is a defensive action initiated by the body to dispose of irritants or injurious agents. Many irritants must come from common foods because when these foods are eliminated from the diet the body will usually halt the inflammatory activity and the arthritis symptoms will subside.

It is far more sensible to help the body remove the irritants which it is trying to destroy with inflammation than it is to take drugs which will stop the inflammatory process. While the drugs may turn off the "fire alarm" of pain, they do not put out the "fire" of the underlying arthritis.

Arthritis is one of the most common afflictions of mankind. There is a way to help arthritis without resorting to drugs with their many side effects. Arthritis can be helped with proper diet and fasting, though it is necessary to be supervised by an experienced doctor. If such a doctor can be found, an arthritic can look forward to many years with very little pain, plus freedom from drugs.

« « « ◯ » » »

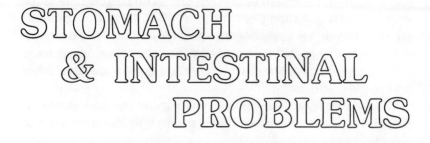

STOMACH & INTESTINAL PROBLEMS

The stomach and intestines give people more problems than almost all the other organs of the body combined. Just one of the problems in this region, peptic ulcers of the stomach, affects up to 10% of the population of this country sometime during life. What with the high incidence of gastritis (stomach inflammation), Crohn's disease (inflammation and ulceration of the small intestines), ulcerative colitis (inflammation and ulceration of the large intestine), irritable colon (pain with diarrhea and/or constipation), simple constipation, and diverticulitis (inflammed pockets in the large intestine), there is probably no one in this country who escapes problems with the digestive system.

If you are astounded at the frequency of these conditions, you will be even more amazed to find out about some of the largely unknown facts regarding treatment of these problems. Peptic ulcers, for instance, have probably been more mistreated than any other health condition. For many years the bland and white "Sippy" diet has been in vogue. This diet consists of plenty of dairy products and soft cooked cereals with almost complete avoidance of fruits and vegetables. Would you believe that this diet has never been proven to be helpful yet it is still commonly used? Sadly, this is the case. Also, it is known that the high fat content of this diet increases the risk of heart disease in ulcer patients by three times.

As if these problems with the "Sippy" diet were not enough, the high protein content of the diet stimulates excessive stomach acid secretion which further worsens the ulcer. The diet itself is extremely acidic which also complicates the situation.

What about the treatment for Crohn's disease and ulcerative

« « « O » » »

colitis? Current treatment consists of drugs and surgery. The list of drugs in use is quite long, but the most powerful one in common use is cortisone. Yet cortisone is so hazardous that if you don't die from Crohn's or colitis, then you may die of cortisone use since it is known to destroy bone, skin, muscle, glands, plus have other serious side effects.

Clearly people are dying for want of a safe plan to follow with digestive system disorders. I will attempt to describe such a program herein.

Instead of using separate names for inflammation and/or ulceration in every different corner of the digestive system, I will discuss the general care of these problems wherever they occur in the entire region. We can then dispense with the following terms: gastritis, peptic ulcer, Crohn's disease, ulcerative colitis, and diverticulitis. Having read the earlier chapters on inflammation and ulceration, you know that these processes are essentially the same wherever they occur.

The health recovery program is almost identical for all cases of inflammation and/or ulceration in the digestive system. Recently, research with Crohn's disease has been published which reveals the success of a dietary program which can be utilized for most digestive tract problems.

In July of 1985 this research was published in the British medical journal *Lancet*. Doctors at the Addenbrooke's Hospital in Cambridge, England, studied the effect of dietary changes with Crohn's disease patients. When you read the results bear in mind that standard medical thinking holds that this condition can only be controlled with powerful drugs and that, even with such therapy, flareups are common, necessitating surgical removal of portions of the small intestine.

Yet the researchers in the *Lancet* found that 70% of patients maintained a healthy small intestine by making simple dietary changes while completely avoiding drugs. The following foods were the most common causes of trouble (listed in decreasing order of severity): wheat, dairy products, cabbage family plants (cabbage, broccoli, cauliflower, brussel sprouts, turnips), corn, yeast, citrus fruits, coffee, lamb, and beef. Foods which none of

« « « ◯ » » »

the patients had problems with included rice, barley, rye, chicken, turkey, banana, and potato.

To detect food intolerances patients were not allowed to eat and could drink nothing but water for approximately one week (most received intravenous feeding). Almost all subjects were free of intestinal symptoms at the end of this week. They were then given one food per day. The foods which caused problems caused immediate flareups and patients were then advised to avoid these foods. By avoiding the aggravating foods, 70% of the patients were symptom-free and taking no drugs at the end of six months.

So that there is no confusion, avoiding wheat products means avoiding white bread, whole wheat bread, spaghetti, macaroni, donuts, most cookies, and the many other foods which contain wheat. The labels on food products must be read carefully since wheat is an ingredient in a wide variety of foods.

Because inflammation and ulceration are the same wherever they occur in the digestive system, the health recovery program for all such conditions is the same as with Crohn's disease. But to ensure success, there are a few additional important guidelines.

Never attempt to treat yourself with a serious problem in the digestive system. You must be under a doctor's care. Fasting, in particular, is only safe if supervised.

After fasting long enough to allow symptoms to disappear, avoid high fiber foods when you start eating. The coarse fiber contained in lettuce, celery, green beans, apples, cereals, and grains can be quite irritating. It is usually necessary at first to cook all fruits, vegetables, and grains in order to soften the fiber. These foods do not need to be cooked to the state of mush, just enough so that they are relatively soft.

After approximately one week of fasting (this time period is variable), the best foods to start on are vegetable soups, mashed bananas, mashed steamed potatoes, applesauce (unsweetened, of course), soft pears, and other such soft fruits and vegetables. After about one week of these foods any grains besides wheat products can be added.

Following one week of fruits, vegetables, and grains, one can

« « « ◯ » » »

add small amounts of blended raw seeds and nuts; or if you cannot remain a vegetarian add chicken, turkey, and fish. The amounts of these foods must be limited to three ounces per day.

Any flare-up in symptoms must be dealt with by either complete fasting or a diet limited to small amounts of cooked fruits and vegetables for at least one week.

With constipation and irritable colon there is no inflammation or ulceration. These conditions are therefore much easier to overcome. A one week fast, followed by the diet described in this chapter and in the back of the book, will almost always solve the problem.

Constipation can be understood quite simply. The digestive tract is limited in the amount of work that it can do, much the same as each of us is limited in the number of miles that we can walk or run. Eating excessive amounts of food will overload the digestive tract and cause exhaustion. Eating excessive amounts of foods that are too concentrated (meats, dairy products, and grains) will also overwork this region. The digestive tract will then have too little energy to complete the elimination process. The solution is a period of rest for the intestines, followed by a more rational diet.

As with all health problems, diet is not everything. The digestive system is especially responsive to emotional upsets. Excessive stress in the form of overwork, worry, anxiety, fear, depression, exhaustion and all other types must be controlled or longterm results will be unsatisfactory. Exercise is quite helpful, as are chiropractic adjustments.

Also, the digestive tract is extremely sensitive to toxic insult in the form of alcohol, coffee, cigarettes, and other such irritants. These substances must be avoided.

What about colonics and enemas? Are they needed to clean out the lower intestine? No. An enema involves running water into the lower intestine (colon) from a small bag hung about two feet above the body. When the colon gets full of water, the person will then evacuate. A colonic is similar, but it is performed by a therapist in a clinic setting. Water is pumped into the colon, then drained out by a tube which remains in the rectum.

« « « ◯ » » »

Enemas and colonics are not needed to clean out the colon because the colon is fully capable of cleansing itself. When the wrong types or amounts of food are no longer eaten, the colon will be able to completely cleanse itself. There is no hardened, caked-on crust of toxic waste materials lining the colon which can only be removed by colonics.

When unhealthy foods are eaten, absorption will take place in the small intestine. Enemas and colonics will not be able to prevent absorption of such foods since they can only wash out the colon which is many feet downstream of the small intestine.

In the digestive system, as in the other areas of the body, the potential for self-healing is great. Simple changes in lifestyle will usually do the job. In this way the tragedy of a lifetime of drugs with their side effects, plus the specter of multiple surgeries, can usually be eliminated.

« « « ○ » » »

SKIN DISEASES

We all want healthy skin, skin that is free of blemishes and is flushed with a healthy pink color. What is the best way to accomplish this? Should we just slap on creams and salves as if we were putting spot remover on a piece of clothing? No. The way to healthy skin is not from outside-in. Rather, it is from inside-out.

The skin is not an inert covering, like a suit of clothes. It is a living, functioning organ. In fact, the skin is the largest organ of the body. The health status, and the resultant beauty, of the skin is a direct reflection of the health status of the body as a whole. Skin problems cannot be "cured" by applying powerful chemicals. But the body can heal skin problems from within when the proper conditions are present.

Skin problems respond beautifully to a healthful lifestyle program. As with all other illnesses, the skin will not develop an illness unless there is a direct cause of the illness. The cause is almost always found in the area of lifestyle: diet, exercise, stress, rest, etc. When the cause is removed, the body will usually completely heal the skin, even if no direct skin treatment in the form of creams and salves has been used.

The relation of skin illnesses to health habits and lack thereof is simple to understand. An unhealthy lifestyle will almost always result in toxemia (see the chapter on this subject). When toxemia is present the body will make every effort possible to eliminate the toxins. The kidneys and liver will attempt to filter and cleanse the blood. The sweat glands of the skin will function in the same mode and help to eliminate toxins from the blood.

Scientists have known for years that sweat glands remove some of the same toxins as do the kidneys. If the kidneys do an incomplete job of eliminating wastes, some of the chemicals which usually appear in the urine will be found on the skin. Urochrome, the chemical that makes urine yellow, is found on the skin of people with kidney failure, giving rise to a characteristic yellow haze that urologists immediately recognize as a sign of

« « « O » » »

severe kidney problems.

Therefore, when toxemia is present, the sweat glands will eliminate toxins through the pores onto the skin. These toxins will often cause an irritation of the skin. Depending upon the individual's predisposition, one of many skin diseases may develop. In some cases viruses and bacteria may proliferate due to the presence of foreign chemicals on the skin. The result may be psoriasis, acne, eczema, urticaria, or others.

When the toxemia is relieved through healthier lifestyle practices, the sweat glands of the skin will cease their elimination activity. The skin irritation will disappear and the viruses and bacteria will no longer grow. Relief of toxemia will lead to remarkably clear and healthy skin.

Remember, skin problems can only be healed from inside-out. Creams and salves will rarely have more than a minor, temporary effect.

A major cause of toxemia is a disturbed emotional state such as chronic anxiety, depression, and fear. Therefore disturbed emotions will result in toxemia and skin problems. But the effect of emotions on the skin is so immediate and dramatic that we can conclude that there is a more direct connection via the nerves besides the chemical effect of toxemia. Any emotional disturbance may cause skin problems in the absence of actual toxemia.

Millions, if not billions, of dollars are spent yearly by consumers trying to produce beautiful skin with one after another allegedly "miracle" cleansers, creams, or salves. What waste of effort! Until junk food is largely eliminated and plenty of wholesome whole foods eaten instead, until an exercise program is followed on a regular basis, until negative emotions are minimized, neither the skin nor any other organ of the body will ever develop good health. Don't give up hope no matter how bad your skin looks. The power of the body to heal itself rarely shows itself as dramatically as when gray, blemished, unhealthy skin becomes pink, clear, and refreshed with a healthful lifestyle program.

« « « ◯ » » »

HEADACHES

Headaches are extremely common. In fact, there are few people who can say that they have never experienced one. An occasional headache is not necessarily cause for concern. But when headaches begin to occur more than once or twice a week and when medication is needed as a remedy, then there is a problem which requires immediate attention.

The worst approach for headaches is to rely on medication. Headaches are a symptom of a deeper problem. Therefore, to solely use drugs to remove the pain will allow the cause of the headaches to remain untreated. It is crucial that the cause of headache pain be identified and eliminated or one's overall health may be threatened.

It is also hazardous to solely rely on medications for headache relief because of the side effects of the drugs. Every headache drug, from aspirin to Inderol, has multiple side effects. These range from stomach irritation and ringing in the ears to kidney and liver failure. Doctors have long known that people who take pain relievers as mild as aspirin for many years risk severe damage to their kidneys and liver.

Fortunately there are alternatives. Most headache problems can be resolved with an improved diet, stress reduction, regular exercise, and chiropractic adjustments. The exceptions are found when headaches result from cancer (brain tumor), meningitis, tuberculosis, or some other extremely serious problem. But these problems are quite rare. Probably less than one in 5,000 headache cases results from one of these conditions.

Most headaches can be divided into one of four categories: vascular (involving the blood vessels), extracranial (resulting from problems in the teeth, sinuses, eyes, or ears), traumatic (commonly the result of auto accidents), and psychological (from stress-induced muscle tension). These four types of headaches respond well to lifestyle changes.

The most common vascular headache is migraine. Not all

« « « O » » »

severe headaches are migraines as is commonly thought. Migraines involve not just head pain, but also nausea, vomiting, sensitivity to light, and occasional dizziness. These headaches can be quite crippling. Yet the solution is often simple. Scientific studies have found that most migraines result from food allergies. The most common provoking foods are dairy products, eggs, chocolate, oranges, wheat, and red wine. Elimination of these foods usually provides a satisfactory solution to migraines.

A major cause of migraines and other vascular headaches is toxemia. When the level of toxins in the body becomes excessively high, the nerves and blood vessels in the head and neck region become irritated. Such irritation can trigger headache pain. The solution is to reduce the level of toxins by careful lifestyle changes. Fasting may be of great benefit.

The second major type of headaches, extracranial, requires attention to the area of the body which is producing the pain. If there is a deep cavity in a tooth, this must be filled to remove the cause of headache pain. Ear and sinus inflammation can cause headache pain. Such inflammation is usually evidence of the body's effort to destroy toxins which have accumulated in these regions. Cooperation with this effort will result in a decrease in inflammation and headache pain.

The third type of headache is traumatic. Following an injury to the head or neck, nerves will often be irritated due to tearing of ligaments, muscles, tendons, and other tissues. Headaches of this type respond well to a gentle chiropractic approach which combines the use of massage, heat, and other physical therapy measures with spinal manipulation to relax muscles, mobilize the bones of the spine, and improve circulation.

The fourth type of headache is psychological. Stress in any form can cause muscle tension which irritates nerves, often resulting in headaches. Chiropractic and physical therapy treatments can be quite helpful in reducing the pain of psychologically caused headaches. But longterm relief will only come from a reduction in stress. The cause of anxiety, depression, worry, fear, or other aggravating emotions must be eliminated or the headaches will continue to recur.

« « « ◯ » » »

Headaches are extremely common and the solution most people seek usually is medication. Yet this habit can be very self-destructive because it leaves the cause of the headache pain untreated, and the drugs which are usually taken have many negative side effects. Fortunately however, headaches can almost always be resolved through simple lifestyle changes including improved nutrition, stress reduction, regular exercise, and chiropractic adjustments.

« « « ◯ » » »

Section Four

HOW TO UNLEASH YOUR BODY'S HEALING POWER

YOUR BODY'S HEALING POWER

Health is the outcome of living more healthfully. Health is built by the body. So-called "cures" relieve symptoms of poor health, but do not build better health. To build health, we must stop doing anything which worsens health, and must also live in such a way that the body will get what it needs to function normally.

Every specialist tends to believe that his specialty is the answer. Nutritionists often believe that if you eat properly, then that is all you will need to achieve perfect health. Many psychologists contend that if you are truly happy, you will be healthy no matter what you eat. Some exercise enthusiasts claim that if you get enough exercise, you will be healthy even if you are miserable. Some would claim that exercise is the ultimate remedy for anxiety and depression.

But such limited viewpoints as those just described are incompatible with true health. To achieve good health it is necessary to work on all areas of life.

Arnold K., a 45 year old man, came to me complaining of chronic fatigue. His medical history showed no serious illnesses, the physical exam uncovered no apparent problems, blood and urine tests were normal, diet and exercise were good. Yet Arnold was very unhappy in his work, had no close friends and was not married. The cause of his fatigue was unhappiness. Without something to be excited and happy about in life, Arnold's body could not muster up the energy needed to function healthfully.

Bill R., a 52 year old man, came in concerned with chest pain. He had seen numerous doctors all of whom had found, after extensive testing, that the blood vessels in his heart were blocked with fat, and he had been told surgery would be needed. Bill could not understand why this happened since he exercised

« « « ◯ » » »

regularly. He was happy at work and at home and he had many good friends, so stress did not seem to be a factor. But when he was asked to write down everything he usually eats, he listed eggs and bacon for breakfast, hamburgers for lunch, salad with fatty dressing and beef for dinner, and ice cream for dessert. The cause of the heart problem was the diet. Even with a good exercise program and a relatively stress-free life, Bill could not be healthy on a high fat diet. When he changed his diet to one high in fruits, vegetables, and grains, and low in meats and dairy products, his heart pain disappeared and he was able to avoid coronary bypass surgery.

Millie B., a 55 year old woman, came in complaining of chronic digestive problems. Gas, bloating, constipation alternating with diarrhea, and indigestion were almost daily occurrences. A careful medical history followed by a complete examination including an X-ray study of the stomach and lower intestine turned up no tumors, ulcers, or inflammation. The diagnosis was irritable bowel syndrome. But, surprisingly, we found that Millie was following a careful diet and was quite happy with her life except for her stomach troubles. When asked if she ever exercised, Millie explained that she was too busy to do so. Since this was the only area of healthful living practice that she did not follow, I recommended that she walk briskly at least 30 minutes every night. After two weeks of this, Millie happily reported that her stomach was giving her no more trouble.

Eating properly is important, but not a cure-all. Reducing stress is essential, but by itself will not solve all health problems. Regular exercise is a requirement of any health-building program, but it will not build good health if it is the only healthful living practice followed.

To be healthy it is essential that every aspect of life be scrutinized and modified. Eating the proper foods, reducing stress, exercising regularly, getting enough rest, drinking pure water, breathing unpolluted air, exposing the skin to the proper amount of sunlight, avoiding accidents and injuries: all are necessary to build health.

We live in a world of dramatic medical interventions. If your

« « « ◯ » » »

hip joint disintegrates, you can have a new one installed. If your heart blood vessels are blocked with fat, you can have them replaced with new clean ones. Do you need to have your lower back checked for a slipped disc? Then have a CAT scan taken with a million dollar machine hooked up to a computer. The glory of high-tech medicine is at hand. The age of bionic bodies is right around the corner. If a body part breaks down, we may be able to purchase a new one.

Next to the shine of the medical/hospital industrial complex, simple changes in lifestyle pale in comparison. But remember that changing the way you live will not cure anything. It is the body that heals. The changes in diet, exercise habits, etc., serve to unleash the internal healing powers of the body. And the functioning of these powers outshine any aspect of high-tech medicine.

In the 20th century we have developed a tremendous respect for the abilities of scientists. Researchers can take a tree apart and study every part down to the smallest molecule. They can say what chemicals are found in a tree, how the tree builds new limbs, the way that nutrients are moved from the ground to the leaves, how the tree reproduces, and everything else to do with it.

But never forget that even though scientists can take a tree apart and reveal many secrets, no scientist can build a tree. Only Mother Nature can produce a living plant or animal.

Nature has programmed into every living thing the ability to heal itself when needed. The mechanisms employed by nature are far more complex than anything used by doctors. When you live more healthfully, you give nature the opportunity to do its work. The results speak for themselves. After following a new way of life, your body will clearly show you from within the power of healing that will build health.

« « « ◯ » » »

HOW TO EAT

I have heard it said that anyone who eats considers himself to be a nutritionist. The subject of food is one that is near and dear to our hearts. To criticize what someone eats is almost the same as criticizing his religion. Eating, then, is a personal affair.

But unfortunately most of us have been taught how to eat by people who really do not teach the healthiest diet. With all due respect to our parents who meant well, the typical American diet passed down through the generations is a nutritional disaster. Authorities have announced to the public that science has connected our daily fare to cancer, heart disease, strokes, diabetes, and many other serious illnesses. So there is no doubt that a change must be made.

How should we eat? From where should we get our information? It is easy to be confused since one year a book comes out telling people to eat a high protein, low carbohydrate diet, then the next year a new book recommends the opposite. One scientist says cholesterol will kill you, then another says that this is unproven. With all this confusion people are tempted to just give up and eat whatever they choose with carefree abandon.

But there is hope. There is a formula for eating which has been scientifically proven to be proper; on which there is 99% agreement among scientists.

Certainly we know that there must be one general eating plan that is right for all human beings. No one will argue that one gorilla should eat a particular diet, while his brother gorilla needs a different diet. All dogs basically eat the same food; all cows eat the same food; in fact, all members of any type of animal species eat the same food. There are slight variations in proportions, but the overall plan is the same. This is also true of human beings.

Food is primarily made of protein, fat, and carbohydrate. Also found are water, vitamins, minerals, and other substances present in minimal amounts. But the major bulk of food is made of protein, fat, and carbohydrate. Therefore, when we discuss any

« « « ◯ » » »

diet, we can define it as being either high or low in protein, high or low in fat, and high or low in carbohydrate. The Atkins and Scarsdale diets are high in protein and fat and low in carbohydrate. The Pritikin and Eat To Win diets are high in carbohydrate and low in protein and fat. So when when we discuss the ideal diet, we must discuss the requirements for carbohydrate, fat, and protein, and the hazards if the wrong types or amounts of these substances are eaten.

It is also necessary to discuss food preparation and refining. There is no use in choosing an ideal type of food and then destroying its nutritional value before we eat it.

The amount of food eaten is important. The ideal types of food, if eaten in too great or too little an amount, can have devastating effects on the health.

The micronutrient content of food is crucial. Besides carbohydrate, fat, and protein, there is a great concern with vitamins and minerals. How much is enough? How much is too much? How can we assure adequate intake with our food choices? Do we need to eat organically grown foods to be sure that enough vitamins are present? Should we take large doses of vitamins and minerals to prevent or treat illnesses?

There are many other important issues: is vegetarianism good or bad for health? Is fiber important and where does it come from? If we cannot control our eating habits, what should we do?

In future chapters, I will attempt to answer these questions with answers that are scientifically documented. But where science has no answers, I will appeal to your common sense. In some cases, logical reasoning is the only path we can follow.

You will find that the eating plan which I recommend is not new. If it were, it would not be valid. Man has been on the earth for thousands of years and the proper diet for his body is the same now as it was in the beginning. The intestines, heart, lungs, blood, arteries, veins, eyes, brain—in fact, all of the body parts—are fundamentally the same today as they were eons ago. Because the human body is unchanged, we know that the proper diet is also the same today as it has always been.

« « « ◯ » » »

HOW MUCH SHOULD WE EAT?

How much food should we eat? This is a very important consideration since even the healthiest food, if eaten in too great an amount, will make us sick.

The amount of food needed is totally individual. Not only is the individual's need unique, but there is great variation from day to day and from meal to meal for each person.

The body is not like a machine that needs the same amount of fuel every day at specific times that never change. Such an imaginary machine, at 8:00 a.m. every day of the year, would need a specific amount of fuel. At 12:00 p.m., the machine would again need a specific amount of fuel. Again at 6:00 p.m. the machine would need its regular dose. The machine never changes. It never increases nor decreases its output. Its needs are always exactly the same.

Most people eat as if they were made like such a machine, eating the same amount of food every day and eating strictly by the clock. Problems result, however, because the human body is nothing like an imaginary machine. Our need for food varies from day to day. The time of day when food should be eaten is always changing. The amount of food needed at each meal changes frequently.

If we eat when the body does not need or want food, we will make ourselves sick sooner or later. Therefore we must determine on a daily and even hourly basis how much we should eat. Does this sound difficult? Maybe, but only because most of us have no such experience. But with a little effort and practice, anyone can master this skill.

We are born with an instinct which compels us to eat when we are truly hungry and refuse food if we are not hungry. But this instinct is usually lost as the years pass. It is customary to eat by

« « « ◯ » » »

the clock: breakfast at 8:00 a.m., lunch at noon, and dinner at 6:00 p.m. Children learn this practice at a young age. If they get to the breakfast table and have no appetite, they are told that a good breakfast is essential for a productive day. If they go to lunch and want to eat lightly, the smell and appearance of processed foods may override this desire. At dinnertime there may again be no appetite due to the large lunch but the child is told to finish everything on his plate because of the starving children in India. After a few years of this type of conditioning, most children will lose touch with the true sensation of hunger.

When sickness strikes, it is common to lose the appetite. This is called anorexia. Don't confuse this with anorexia nervosa which is a loss of food desire due to an emotional disturbance. When someone has a cold or the flu, it is normal to want to avoid food.

But what are we told when we are sick and have no appetite? That we must eat or we will never recover our strength. So even though the sight of food, not too mention the taste, is repulsive, we force some food down the hatch.

The problem that results from such typical eating practices is sickness. When the body says that it wants no food, and we jam food in anyway, we are sowing the seeds of illness. The body can only handle a certain limited amount of food and it signals the brain that enough has been eaten by turning off the appetite. When we disregard this message, we give the body an excess of food which leads to a whole host of problems.

Overloading the body with food is a cause of overweight, a major cause of diabetes, high blood pressure, and other conditions. Heart disease and strokes result when we eat too many high cholesterol foods; cancer when we eat too many high fat foods; and accelerated aging when we eat too much of any type of food. When we are sick and overeat, there will usually be a prolongation and worsening of the illness. Clearly, overeating damages health.

How much should we eat? To know, we must tune into the messages coming from within the body. This does not mean that every time the stomach growls, we should eat. When there is a feeling of distress in the belly, many people stuff food down as

« « « ◯ » » »

fast as possible. But this is no more healthful than giving an addict a fix. True hunger is not a distressing sensation.

Learn to recognize hunger as a comfortable but compelling desire for food. You may have to miss a few meals in order to discover how to recognize hunger. Most of us have never gone without food long enough to give the sensation of hunger a chance to emerge.

When symptoms of distress develop after a person has gone without food for a number of hours, this is not a good sign and does not mean that food should be immediately eaten. If a coffee addict gets a headache when he doesn't get enough coffee, would we advise him to solve the problem by having another cup? If a heroin addict has the shakes when he has gone too long without a fix, would we advise him to quickly get an injection? Of course not. Yet this is what we do with food. Many of the foods we eat create the same type of situation in the body as do coffee, heroin and other addictive substances. When we have distress from not eating, we should not eat until the distress vanishes.

This may take an hour, a day, or even two or three days, but we must learn to hang in there and wait it out. I strongly advise that you have a knowledgeable doctor available to help you through this process. But when you have struggled with the discomfort of not eating long enough to begin to feel good, you will discover true hunger and eating will lead to health, not disease.

Once you are in touch with true hunger, follow it wherever it leads you. If you are not hungry when you wake up in the morning, don't eat. If the next day you are hungry, then eat. If you come home from work at night exhausted and with little appetite, skip dinner. If you have just had a fight with someone and feel upset, don't eat until you calm down. When you are sick and have no appetite, don't eat until hunger returns.

You will not lose strength if you don't eat when you are not hungry. You will not fail to recover strength if you don't eat when you are sick. In fact, by doing what the body wants you to do, you will become much healthier than before.

The general rules of how much to eat and when to eat are:

« « « ◯ » » »

only eat when you are truly hungry; stop eating immediately after your hunger has been satisfied; never eat when you are upset, exhausted, or sick; do not eat immediately before or after intense exercise. It is imperative that these rules be followed or even the healthiest food will lead to illness.

PROTEIN

One would think that "protein" is the name of a religion, not a nutrient, based on the way people talk about it. It is common to hear that protein is a miracle food which will solve all problems. But is protein such a wonder food? Do we need to work hard to ensure adequate protein intake?

The truth is that protein is no wonder food. It is easy to get enough from the diet, and most people eat far too much and damage their health.

Why the great protein mania? Because of clever advertising campaigns waged by the meat, dairy, and egg industries. Why do people buy the cars that they do? Because the car manufacturers have invested millions to create the desire for their product. Why do people dress the way they do? Because the clothing industry has created a passion for the new style. The same is true with protein.

The meat industry has most people convinced that meat is essential for strength and that it is a sign of "high class" to eat steak many times a week. The diary and egg industries have convinced the public that the protein in milk and eggs is crucial for good health. Most people would be genuinely frightened at the idea of a diet without meat, dairy foods, and eggs.

But what are the facts? If you talk to scientists who have PhD's in nutrition or biochemistry, you will uncover the truth. It is, in fact, easy to get enough protein. Meat, dairy products, and eggs are not required for good health. Most people eat too much protein and their health suffers as a result.

The Recommended Daily Allowance (RDA) for protein is about 50 grams per day. Yet statistics show that the average American eats 100 grams per day. Clearly, most people eat twice as much protein as they need.

But there is more to this story: the RDA figure of 50 grams includes a large safety margin. Scientists have found that the true need is closer to 25 grams.

« « « ◯ » » »

There have been many studies in which subjects have been fed 20—25 grams of protein per day. Patients with kidney failure, heart failure, coronary artery disease, and high blood pressure have eaten such a low protein diet and their health improved. Doctors measured blood levels of protein, amino acids (subunits of protein), and hemoglobin (made of protein) and all remained normal on 20—25 grams of protein per day.

Will stress increase the need for protein? If so, since we live in a high stress society, should we eat a larger amount of protein to compensate? No. Scientific research has found that stress does not significantly increase the protein need. Studies found that the nervous tension of final exams and of sleep deprivation increased the need for protein by only one gram or less per day.

But don't athletes need more protein? Weightlifters are especially concerned. The myth that athletes need more protein was formulated in the 1800s and disproved in 1866, but health spa counselors still hang on to their passion for protein. Dozens of studies have proven that heavy work and/or exercise will not increase the need for protein. When people are extremely active they need more calories. Calories are to the body what gasoline is to the car; protein is to the body what the engine is to the car. When you drive further at higher speeds, you need more gasoline, not more engines. It is unfortunate that the "more protein makes more muscle" myth is still around when the scientific community has rejected it for decades.

What is protein used for in the body? It is used to build tissue, make hormones and enzymes, hemoglobin and antibodies. So, obviously, sufficient protein intake is crucial. But this is quite easy to accomplish.

Protein deficiency is extremely rare. In fact, it is almost unknown outside of the Third World. The only way to become deficient in protein is to either starve or exclusively eat foods that contain no protein (sugar or oil). If a person eats enough food to maintain near normal weight, and if a variety of whole foods are eaten, a protein deficiency is impossible.

Even in the Third World, a true protein deficiency is rare. It is more common to find a protein-calorie deficiency. The body's primary need is for calories, not for protein. Calories are needed to provide fuel for the heart, lungs, kidneys, and other vital organs. Protein is primarily needed for building tissue. When there is too little food, the body will need to use all of the food for calorie production. Therefore the body will convert the protein in the food to calories. This is a very inefficient process and will only occur when a person is near starvation. For this reason the term "protein-calorie deficiency" is used. If the starving person had enough food to eat, even if the food were low in protein, there would be no problem since the body would utilize the fats and carbohydrates for calorie production and spare the protein for tissue building purposes.

Many people believe that meat, dairy foods, and eggs are the only sources of protein. But this is not true since all whole foods contain protein. A banana and a pear each provide one gram; a stalk of broccoli, six grams; an avocado, four grams; a carrot, one gram. Breads and cereals have significant amounts: one slice of bread has 2 to 3 grams, one cup of cereal has 2 grams. Foods like nuts, seeds, and beans are loaded: ½ cup of almonds has 13 grams, ½ cup of dried beans has 7 to 8 grams. By comparison, three ounces of steak contains 24 grams of protein, one egg 6 grams, one ounce of cheese 7 grams.

Meats, dairy foods, and eggs are rich in protein. But, if enough of all the other foods are eaten so that normal weight is maintained and if animal foods are not used, there would still be more protein than needed. A daily diet of three to four fruits, a large vegetable salad, two servings of grains, and three ounces of nuts or beans would easily provide 35 grams of protein per day. Since the need is for 20 to 25 grams, there would be more than enough.

What about the quality of protein? Are meat, dairy, and egg proteins the only ones "complete" enough to support good health? No. Protein quality is rated in percents: egg is 94%, cheese 82%, meat and poultry 67%, fish 80%, grains and cereals 50 to 70%, vegetables about 82%, legumes, nuts, and seeds 40 to 60%. But you don't have to eat perfect 100% proteins to rebuild body tissue. If a protein of 50% quality is eaten, you would just need to consume twice as much as you would of a 100% quality protein to

« « « ◯ » » »

get the same amount of usable protein. Therefore meat, dairy, and egg protein need not be eaten to ensure adequate protein nutrition.

Do you need to combine lower quality proteins together at each meal so that one protein makes up for the deficiencies in the other protein? No. The body maintains a large pool of the subunits of protein, the amino acids. Therefore if a protein is eaten which is too low in certain amino acids, the body can supplement the protein from its reservoir of amino acids and make this protein relatively complete and usable.

Again, it is important to repeat that it would take an incredible amount of imagination and planning to develop a protein deficiency. It is easy to get enough. Except in cases of starvation, kidney or liver failure, cancer or another type of severe disease, protein deficiency is not found. We must overcome the paranoia created by the meat and dairy industries and learn to eat rational amounts of protein.

Should we eat extra protein to provide a margin or safety? If some is good, more must be better. But this is a dangerous philosophy since even water, if consumed in too large an amount, can be deadly. Protein can cause serious health problems if eaten in excess.

One danger from excess protein intake is increased deposits of fat on the walls of blood vessels, causing heart attacks and strokes. Dr. Kilmer McCully, professor of pathology at Harvard Medical School, has proven this connection. Excessive intake of protein supplies excessive amounts of methionine, one of the animo acids. Methionine is broken down into homocysteine which irritates the walls of blood vessels. This irritation causes fat deposits.

Too much protein can also accelerate the aging process. Dr. Charles Barrows of the National Institute of Aging has done many experiments which have documented this hazard. A high protein intake results in excessive utilization of cellular "machinery," thereby causing premature aging.

Excess protein has been shown to increase the amount of calcium lost from the body in the urine. Many researchers believe

« « « O » » »

that a high protein intake may cause osteoporosis by leaching calcium out of the body. In the book *Recommended Dietary Allowances*, it is clearly stated that high levels of protein in the diet greatly increase the need for calcium. Unfortunately, however, most people do not eat enough calcium-rich foods to compensate for the high protein intake.

There is no magic to protein. It is a nutrient that is needed to have a normal, healthy body, but it accomplishes no miracles. We need to become less concerned about getting enough protein because the real problem is a dangerously high intake of protein which contributes to many serious illnesses.

« « « ○ » » »

FAT

Fat in food makes a meal feel like it sticks to your ribs. Fat has a rich flavor and it leaves the stomach feeling full for a long time. We crave fat in food because of its ability to produce deep satisfaction from a meal.

But this craving for fat can be disastrous to your health. Overeating fatty foods results in many types of cancer, heart disease, strokes, plus overweight which contributes to many other diseases, such as diabetes.

The American Heart Association, National Cancer Institute, American Cancer Society, and many other public health and research institutes have called for a reduction in the fat content of the diet. It is rare to find such widespread agreement about diet, but with fat this is the case.

Foods high in fat include meats, dairy products, eggs, nuts, seeds, oils, margarine, mayonaisse, most salad dressings, coconut, avocado, and olives. There are generally two types of fatty foods: those containing saturated fat (animal foods) and those containing unsaturated fat (vegetable foods).

The scientific community is now completely convinced that a high intake of saturated fats will cause a buildup of fat in blood vessels, leading to heart disease and stroke. The foods high in saturated fats are also hazardous because they are loaded with cholesterol. Occasionally you may hear it said that fat has not been proven to be linked to heart disease. But when 99% of scientists agree that fat is a danger, and only 1% say the opposite, the better part of discretion is to go with the majority.

Researchers are also completely convinced that a high fat intake is linked to cancer, especially of the colon, breast, and prostate. Both saturated and unsaturated fats are implicated. Recently the American Cancer Society began a public health advertising campaign to convince people to reduce fat intake.

A high fat diet has an overall negative impact on health. In one study, scientists examined the blood vessels which can be

« « « O » » »

seen in the back of the eye. A fifty power microscope was used so that actual blood cells could be seen floating along inside the blood vessels. When the person ate a meal high in fat, the blood flow slowed considerably, the blood cells became sticky and they clumped together. This reduced the ability of the blood to carry oxygen from the lungs to all internal tissues. Since the people who participated in this study already had restricted blood flow to the heart, they developed heart pain from oxygen starvation when the blood flow slowed and the cells clumped.

When we speak of supplying nutrients to the cells, we usually ignore the most important nutrient, one which we cannot live without for more than three minutes. This nutrient is oxygen. But breathing air is not enough to ensure adequate oxygen supply to the cells. We require a healthy transport system. If a person eats too much fat, this transport system will become considerably less effective, leading to significant oxygen starvation. Every part of the body will suffer when the ideal amount of oxygen is not delivered. In fact, heart attacks and strokes result when oxygen starvation kills heart and brain cells. And some researchers believe that chronic oxygen deprivation may make normal body cells become cancerous.

Another problem with fat is its caloric density. Caloric density means the number of calories per pound of food. Vegetables have the lowest caloric density. One pound of celery contains only 52 calories. But cheese, a food high in fat, contains close to 2000 calories per pound. If you fill up on vegetables, you can feel satisfied and have eaten only a few hundred calories. If you fill up on high fat food, it is easy to eat over one thousand calories before your stomach feels full. In a country where overweight is a major problem, it is important to eat foods of lower caloric density to keep the weight down.

Imagine a large vegetable salad with red ripe tomatoes, deep green Boston lettuce, carrot, celery, cucumber, red bell pepper, and fresh peas. Total calories: about 200. A highly nutritious meal, low in fat, high in fiber, consistent with all health principles. But then comes the high fat salad dressing: two tablespoons of blue cheese dressing, containing over 200 calories of fat. Such a

« « « ◯ » » »

dressing turns a healthful salad into a high fat disaster.

When you first switch from a high fat to a low fat diet, you may feel uncomfortable for about a month. Fat in the stomach makes the stomach retain food for a longer time, thereby making a person feel full longer. When the stomach has been accustomed to a high fat diet and then the dietary fat level is greatly reduced, the stomach will empty very rapidly and the person will say that he never feels full. But after about one month on a low fat diet, the stomach will adjust and not empty as rapidly. Therefore the feeling of fullness after a meal will last longer and the shift to the new diet will become easier.

The American tradition of diet is one high in fat. The usual percentage of calories in the diet coming from fat is 40%. The most conservative authorities have recommended that this be reduced to 30% (American Heart Association), whereas the most radical nutritionists have recommended a 10% fat diet (Pritikin). The conclusion from reviewing many such recommendations is that 20 to 25% is a safe figure.

But, in considering dietary fats, it is crucial to discuss the type of fat and the way it has been processed and/or cooked. The oil in a sesame seed is totally different from the oil in a bottle of sesame seed oil. Processed oils are treated five times with very high levels of heat, plus many other destructive types of manipulations. Processing destroys the food factors found in the sesame seed which nature provides to aid in the digestion and utilization of the oil. The conclusion is that the healthiest fats are those found in the unprocessed natural state.

As the years pass, scientists are continually amazed at the handiwork of nature. Foods produced by nature are in the healthiest form if they are processed only by the teeth. Nothing good is added when foods are extracted, refined, processed, stored, cooked, concentrated, transformed, and manipulated in many other ways. You can be sure that health value is almost always reduced through such interventions.

Therefore, the best fats to use are avocados, nuts, seeds; and if you cannot be vegetarian, chicken, and fish. Always choose the most natural form of the food (raw, not roasted nuts), the lowest

« « « ◯ » » »

fat content available (trout, not shrimp), and the most conservative method of cooking (never fry). Eat no more than 4 to 5 ounces of high fat food per day (the amount found in ¼ pound of cheese, for example).

Don't ever be concerned about getting too little fat from your diet. The only nutritional need is for the type of fat called essential fatty acids. Scientists have never found a case of dietary deficiency of these substances. They are found in many foods.

Also, you don't need to eat more fat if your skin is dry. The liver can create fat out of carbohydrate and protein. Therefore if the body needs more fat and you are not eating much, the liver will produce some.

To be healthy, avoid a high fat diet. The change to a lower fat intake may be difficult for some people in the beginning, but the reduced risk of heart disease and cancer makes such a change worthwhile. After a few months on the new program, you will not even miss the previous high fat intake.

« « « ◯ » » »

CARBOHYDRATE

Food is primarily made of fat, protein, and carbohydrate. In previous chapters I have recommended that fat and protein intake be greatly reduced. Since carbohydrate is the only remaining major food component, it is therefore necessary to increase its consumption.

What is carbohydrate? This technical word can be translated into the words "sugar" and "starch." "Sugar" encompasses the world of sweets: candy, ice cream, soda pop, honey, fruit juice, carrot juice, fructose, white sugar, molasses, brown sugar, dried fruit, and any other extremely sweet foods. People selling honey will tell you that it is a health food compared to the poison white sugar. People selling fructose, brown sugar, juices, and other sweets will oftentimes say the same. But don't believe it for a minute. Nutritionally there is absolutely no meaningful difference between all the above mentioned sugars.

The word "starch" describes the other major type of carbohydrate. Bread, rice, oatmeal, millet, potatoes, corn, squash, carrots, and all other grains and vegetables contain starch.

Why, if starch consists of sugars, is starch healthful and sugar not? Because when you eat sugar, it is in such a simple form that the body will rapidly absorb it with no delay. This causes the blood sugar level to shoot up, which causes the blood insulin level to rise rapidly. These quick changes produce negative changes in the body, such as hypoglycemia.

But when starch is eaten, it takes a few hours for the body to digest it. One sugar at a time is broken off from the end of the long chain of sugars. Therefore there is only a slow trickle of sugar into the bloodstream, not a flood as occurs when sweets are ingested. The body can gracefully handle such a slow trickle.

Grains, such as bread, and vegetables are starchy foods. Fruit is the other major type of carbohydrate food. Earlier I stated that fruit juice is as sugar-rich as candy, and that candy causes problems for the body. But this is not the case with fruit. Although fruit does contain sugar and no starch, the sugar in fruit is in very

« « « ◯ » » »

low concentration since fruit is mostly water. Also, the sugar in a whole fruit is bonded to fiber. It takes a while for the body to break the sugar off from the fruit fiber so, as with starch, there is no flood of sugar into the bloodstream.

One study measured the result from eating whole apples versus blended apples, versus apple juice. When the whole apples were eaten the blood sugar level gradually increased over a few hours, then it gradually decreased. When the blended apples were eaten the blood sugar level rose much more rapidly and declined more rapidly. When the apple juice was ingested the blood sugar level shot up very fast and then plummeted swiftly. Researchers concluded that blending and juicing released the fruit sugar from the fiber in the fruit, thereby allowing faster absorption into the bloodstream. To the body therefore fruit juice is not much different than candy.

The word "carbohydrate" often conveys a negative connotation. This is because most people, when they hear this word only think of refined carbohydrates such as cake, candy, soda pop, ice cream, white bread, donuts, white sugar, pastries and others. But there is a world of difference between refined and unrefined carbohydrates, so much so that the former is hazardous to your health while the latter forms the major bulk of a healthful diet.

There are many reasons that refined carbohydates (white flour and white sugar) are detrimental to your health. First of all, sugar is a major cause of overweight. It is a food with high caloric density, as is fat. You would need to eat thirty to forty more ounces of vegetables than ounces of sugar to get the same amount of calories.

For the number of calories supplied, sugar gives little feeling of fullness. Thus you eat more and overdose on calories. The overweight which results increases the risk of heart disease, strokes, cancer, diabetes, and many other diseases.

Second, sugar and white flour are devoid of the vitamins and minerals needed for the body to burn these foods to create energy. Therefore the body must draw upon its reserves of vitamins and minerals when sugar and white flour are eaten. If too much of these foods is eaten for too long a time, vitamin and

« « « ◯ » » »

mineral deficiences will inevitably occur.

Third, sugar causes tooth decay. This is a serious health problem which leads to complete loss of teeth by many Americans in later years of life. This loss, besides being of cosmetic and financial concern, also causes nutritional problems because it becomes difficult to eat healthful raw vegetables.

Fourth, sugar requires little digestion so it moves easily and rapidly into the bloodstream. This rush of sugar causes the blood sugar level to rise rapidly. In response to this, the pancreas secretes large amounts of insulin. This causes increased amounts of fat to be deposited on the walls of the blood vessels. These fat deposits are the basic cause of heart disease and strokes and one cause of high blood pressure.

The rapid increase in levels of blood sugar and insulin also may result in an excessive drop in blood sugar levels, resulting in hypoglycemia. In some people symptoms such as fatigue, shaking, depression, headaches, and weakness may occur.

Fifth, sugar is converted by the liver into a type of fat called triglycerides. High levels of this substance in the bloodstream are another cause of heart attacks, strokes, and high blood pressure.

Sixth, when the rush of sugar enters the bloodstream from the digestive tract, scientific studies show that white blood cells are affected. These cells destroy bacteria and digest waste material. The high levels of sugar effectively paralyze white blood cells for a temporary period of time. Therefore if you eat candy when you have an infection, you may prolong the recovery time.

Seventh, sugar and white flour are devoid of fiber. Fiber deficiency leads to colon and rectal cancer, high blood cholesterol levels, hemorrhoids, varicose veins, and many other diseases.

Sugar and white flour, and foods containing these substances, should be avoided, Also, one should limit intake of fruit juices, dried fruits, honey, carrot juice and all other super-sweet foods as there is no significant difference between such foods and pure white sugar.

The good carbohydrates, however, should constitute most of the diet. Whole fruits, vegetables, and grains are the true health

« « « ◯ » » »

foods. They are low in fat, moderate in protein, and high in carbohydrates. They are loaded with the most natural form of vitamins and minerals. Much of the bulk is healthful fiber. You can eat almost unlimited amounts of these foods. But if you tend towards overweight, eat more vegetables and less fruits and grains. If you need to gain weight, do the opposite.

In today's world, the word "protein" has a positive connotation to it whereas the word "carbohydrate" is thought of negatively. We need a major change in thinking: protein should be removed from its pedestal and unrefined carbohydrates put in its place. The high protein foods should be eaten in moderation, while the natural unprocessed carbohydrates should be used liberally. The refined and processed carbohydrates, white sugar and white flour, should be largely avoided since they have many deleterious effects on health.

« « « ◯ » » »

FOOD PROCESSING

The subject of food processing includes all forms of cooking and refining of food. When a food is harvested from the earth it is totally unprocessed. Before most foods are eaten by human beings, some type of processing usually occurs. It is important to discuss the impact of processing on the nutritional value of food.

The only creatures on earth that process food are human beings. No one has ever come upon an animal in the wild cooking food over a fire. Every form of life on earth besides human beings exists exclusively on raw foods. For many years, many health teachers have advocated unprocessed, raw food. What are the scientific facts? Is health endangered by the processing of food?

The answer is yes. Thousands of experiments have proven that food processing significantly reduces the nutritional value of food. But what about nutrients that are yet undiscovered? What is the impact of processing on these unknown factors? If such factors are destroyed, how can we replace them with food supplements? Obviously we cannot replace what we have not identified. Therefore even if we replace all the nutrients *known* to be destroyed by food processing, some of the health-supporting value of food may still be absent.

The only safe course is to eat most foods in the unprocessed form, just as they were created by nature. In fifty years, when scientists discover other necessary nutrients which are destroyed by food processing, those who have eaten foods in the natural state will have no regrets. They will have remained well-nourished by depending on nature, not on modern science.

When food is processed there is generally a 15% loss of minerals, carbohydrates, fats, protein, vitamins K and B3 (niacin). A huge loss of vitamins B1 (thiamine) and C occurrs in food processing; vitamins A, D, E, B6, B12, B2 (riboflavin), pantothenic

« « « ○ » » »

acid, and folacin also suffer great losses.

When unrefined wheat is processed into white flour, 70 to 80% of over forty nutrients are lost. When flour is enriched only three to four nutrients are added. Therefore refined grains have the distinction of being the most depleted of all foods by methods of processing.

Generally the more water used in cooking, the greater the loss of vitamins. Boiling can cause up to 65% loss of vitamin C, whereas waterless cooking causes only a 30% loss. The effects of microwave cooking are similar to those of steaming. When foods are cooked in water, minerals in the food can be leached out. If the cooking water is not used the minerals are lost. Unfortunately there are no exact data as to the amount of minerals lost.

Cooking is known to reduce the availability of minerals to the body. A mineral that becomes less available may be less easily absorbed and/or utilized by the body.

Vitamins C and B1 are easily destroyed by heat. Vitamins A, D, E, B6, B12, riboflavin (B2), pantothenic acid, and folacin are more stable than vitamins C and B1, and so an average loss of 20% can be expected from cooking.

Protein is damaged by heat. Amino acids are the subunits of protein and studies have found that cooking can destroy 5 to 17% of some of the most important amino acids.

Studies on the effects of food processing clearly show many losses of nutrients. Scientists know that processing-related changes in the three-dimensional form of food and in the chemical nature of food will reduce the amount of nutrients available to the body. But since the details are largely unknown it is risky to depend upon processed foods for good nutrition. Be safe rather than sorry: eat most of your food in the raw, unrefined state.

Studying living beings is another approach to evaluating the effect of food processing on health. In clinical practice, a doctor can feed patients raw food exclusively and evaluate the results. In the United States there is a 150 year old tradition of prescribing raw food diets to sick people. Raw foods have been found to be considerably more effective than cooked foods in building and

« « « ◯ » » »

maintaining good health.

A landmark study was done by Dr. Francis Pottenger in the late 1940s, and the findings were published in a major scientific journal. Dr. Pottenger experimented with diet changes using hundreds of cats. Some cats were fed raw meat and raw milk, while others were fed the same meat and milk in the cooked form. The differences between the groups of cats were dramatic.

In the cooked food group miscarriages were common, internal organ and bone structure were abnormal, reproduction failed after a few generations, and behavior was irritable. In the raw food group miscarriages were rare, organ and bone structure was totally normal, reproduction was healthy and normal, and behavior was calm. This study was so carefully designed that we can be sure that the only cause of illness in the cooked food animals was the destruction of health-giving properties in the food from cooking.

Choosing the proper type of food is important. but it is equally important to assure that the nutritional value is not destroyed by processing. The safest path to follow is to eat 75% of your food in the raw, unprocessed form. And if you are ill and attempting to rebuild health, eat 100% of your food raw for at least one month.

In some cases supervision by a doctor will be necessary when the change is made from a cooked food diet to one high in raw foods, because the fiber in raw food can be irritating to the digestive tract, such as in people with a history of stomach ulcer or ulcerative colitis. In most people, eating mostly raw food will improve health dramatically; but if you experience any disturbing symptoms at any time, see your doctor.

« « « ○ » » »

FASTING

It is commonly believed that going without food for more than a day or two is harmful for your health. Since most people feel sick after missing one or two meals, they conclude that a longer fast would be devastating.

But nothing could be further from the truth. Fasting for one to two weeks, a common practice in European countries, is safe, easy after the first day or two, and good for your health.

The idea that fasting improves health is hardly new. Fasting was in vogue in the early days of recorded history. Socrates, Plato, Pthagoras, Hippocrates, Parcelsus, and others recommended fasting to clear the mind and improve health.

Fasting has been studied in depth by scientists since 1900. Also fasting has been used by many doctors in health retreats since the mid-1800's. I interned in one such fasting retreat for six months in 1980, and saw over 1000 people fast for five to twenty-five days at a time.

Fasting can be safe and beneficial, but only when an experienced doctor is available for supervision. Such a doctor can determine whether or not a fast will be safe, how long a person should fast, and when the fast must be broken. The horror stories of fasting result from unsupervised fasts.

Fasting is not a cure. When a person is ill the body simply works overtime to heal itself. Fasting provides an opportunity for the body to heal itself more rapidly and completely than when one is eating.

Many health problems are the result of toxemia. Toxemia is the accumulation of either a substance which is toxic in any amount (lead, mercury, etc.), or a substance which is non-toxic in normal amounts but toxic when in excess (cholesterol). During a fast, the body must live on accumulated materials in the tissues and blood. The body first will utilize the least essential materials present such as excess fat and toxins. As the level of fats and toxins is reduced, improved health will emerge. The previous

« « « ◯ » » »

chapter on toxemia discusses this subject in greater depth.

Studies of fasting have proven that the body prefers to burn non-essential substances like fat long before it will burn the protein of muscle. There are documented cases of obese people fasting 249 days in one case and 382 days in another, with beneficial results.

Studies have found hunger usually disappears after the first two to five days of fasting and that fasting is generally not difficult. One scientist wrote that "the most surprising aspect of this study was the ease with which the prolonged fast was tolerated." Another noted that many patients "reported a marked sense of well-being, suggesting a mild euphoria." The first day or two of fasting can be difficult as patients may develop headaches, nausea, weakness, and muscle pain. But these symptoms rapidly disappear and the patient then becomes comfortable.

When should fasting be employed? Fasting is highly effective in cardiovascular diseases. Most heart attacks and strokes occur because fat deposits in blood vessels block blood flow. Fasting gives the body an opportunity to dissolve these deposits, thereby eliminating the need for coronary bypass surgery.

Scientists have long known that a tremendous amount of salt and water are eliminated from the body during a fast. This causes the blood pressure to go down. After a fast, most people with high blood pressure will be able to stop taking medicine.

Inflammatory diseases such as arthritis, colitis, gastritis, tonsil-litis, and others result from a buildup of toxins in the involved tissue. The body activates the inflammatory process to destroy such toxins. During a fast the body becomes much more efficient in dealing with toxins. As the toxin level decreases, the body will reduce the inflammatory activity and healing will occur. For more information on inflammation, refer to the chapter on that subject.

There are many illnesses which are characterized by sneezing, coughing, a flow of mucous from the nose, vomiting, diarrhea and other such symptoms of elimination of wastes from the body. The most frequent such illnesses are the common cold and the flu. Most people have no appetite when they suffer from such sicknesses. If this loss of appetite is respected and one fasts,

« « « 〇 » » »

the body will be able to burn up and eliminate waste materials far more rapidly than if one eats. When the wastes are eliminated, the body will turn off the sneezing, coughing, vomiting, etc, and one will feel well.

Fasting is of little help with cancer. Actually, if a cancer patient fasts, he may die more quickly. A cancer is like a parasite living off the body's internal tissues. When no food is eaten, the cancer will consume even more of the tissues. This may cause an earlier death.

With benign tumors such as uterine fibroids the story is different. These tumors are not cancers. When a person fasts, the body will break down and destroy such tumors in the same way that it consumes other nonessential tissues and waste products.

Fasting has often been used for weight loss, but it is of no help. When fasting, there is a decrease in the overall rate of internal body activities (metabolism). After a fast the body will burn less calories than before the fast. The body's metabolic rate will remain slower for a long period of time. Therefore if a person begins to eat the same number of calories after the fast as he did before, more weight will be gained than if the same amount of food were eaten before the fast. This is obviously not helpful in a weight loss program.

There are many diseases which have not been discussed in relation to fasting. Can fasting help these conditions? The answer is often yes. Remember that all healing is done by the body. During a fast, the body becomes more efficient at healing because it no longer must expend all its energies in digesting and utilization of food. Therefore most illnesses are resolved more rapidly and completely when fasting is employed. Doctors who specialize in fasting will be able to advise if it will be helpful in a particular case.

In actual practice fasting consists of a diet of only distilled water. Juices are foods and not used during a fast. A successful fast requires plenty of rest. One cannot work and fast. Also, one cannot fast and care for a family, exercise, write a thesis, read two novels per day, argue, or be involved in any other stressful activity. If the supervising doctor permits it, a short walk may be taken.

« « « ◯ » » »

Napping should be one of the major activities of the day. The amount of time that one should fast is totally individual. A person on medication or someone who is in frail health from a recent heart attack, stroke, or other extremely serious illness should not fast at all. If a person is overweight he can fast longer than someone who is underweight. It is best not to fast more than three days without professional supervision. But if one travels to a professional fasting retreat a fast of a few weeks may be safely undertaken.

Breaking a fast in the proper way is crucial. There have been rare instances of severe illness in people who have eaten incorrectly immediately after a long fast. The way to break a fast depends on the length of the fast. A five day fast should be broken with diluted fruit juice (one half juice, one half water) for breakfast, one piece of fruit for lunch and another for dinner. The following day, two fruits for breakfast, a vegetable salad for lunch, and raw and cooked vegetables for dinner. Following this, the normal diet may be resumed.

A fast of twenty days should be broken with two to three days of diluted fruit juice alternating with vegetable juice (a combination of green vegetable and carrot juice). Two days of small meals of raw fruits and vegetables should follow. After this period, nuts, seeds, rice, bread, fish or chicken (if not contaminated by pesticides or other pollutants) can be used. Ten days after the completion of a twenty day fast, a normal diet may be resumed.

Fasting is not a panacea for all health problems. But when properly supervised and conducted, fasting can lead to dramatic health improvements. Study and investigate fasting and consider trying it if dietary changes, exercise programs, and other such measures have not led to sufficient health improvement.

« « « 〇 » » »

VEGETARIANISM

In recent years a great interest in vegetarian diets has emerged. Some people are concerned with the high fat and cholesterol content of meat. Others feel that raising animals for food is cruel and that for this reason they should avoid meat. Because there is so much interest in vegetarianism, it is important to discuss the possible advantages and potential hazards associated with such a dietary change. Fortunately dozens of studies have been done on vegetarians so it is possible to state the facts.

All vegetarians are not the same. While all eat no meat, including fish and chicken, some do use eggs and dairy products; they are termed lacto-ovo-vegetarians. Others use dairy products but no eggs; they are termed lacto-vegetarians. The most strict vegetarians use no eggs or dairy products and are called vegans.

At least seven major studies have evaluated the health of vegetarians of all three classes. Researchers from the Loma Linda School of Medicine, the Harvard School of Public Health, the London Office of Health Economics, the Kingston Hospital in England, and other major scientific centers have taken complete medical histories and performed thorough physical and laboratory examinations. No health problems associated with diet were found. Vegetarians were found to be at least as healthy and, in some of the studies, more healthy than meat-eaters.

Many studies have found that vegetarians are less likely to be overweight than the average person. This is good since lower body weight reduces the risk of cardiovascular diseases, many types of cancer, diabetes, kidney and liver diseases, lung pathology, and problems in pregnancy and childbirth. Also, vegetarians consistently have been found to have lower blood cholesterol levels. This is responsible for a lower risk of heart attacks and strokes.

A vegetarian diet is much higher in fiber than the average diet. One study found that lacto-ovo-vegetarians consumed twice as

« « « ◯ » » »

much, and vegans four times as much fiber as non-vegetarians. A high fiber diet reduces the risk of diverticular disease of the colon, appendicitis, cancer of the colon and rectum, hiatus hernia, hemorrhoids, and varicose veins.

With a vegetarian diet one avoids the harmful chemicals that are sometimes found in meat. In 1979 the General Accounting Office of the U.S. Government reported that 14% of meat in supermarkets contains illegal and potentially harmful residues of animal drugs, pesticides, and environmental contaminants. Of 143 chemicals likely to be found, "forty-two are known to cause or are suspected of causing cancer; twenty of causing birth defects; and six of causing mutations."

The American Dietetic Association reviewed all the studies on vegetarianism with the conclusion that "well-planned vegetarian diets are consistent with good nutritional status."

Frequently people will say: "A vegetarian diet can be healthful but you must be careful in planning." The implication is that if one eats meat then he does not need to be careful in planning his diet but in a meat-less diet caution is necessary. The fact is that caution is always needed in diet planning, whether meat is eaten or not. There is no greater need for caution with a vegetarian diet.

Is meat protein so unique and special that one cannot be healthy without it? Absolutely not. From where does steak get its protein? The grass which the cow eats. The same protein is directly available to human beings from green vegetables and other vegetarian proteins.

Protein is made of amino acids. There are twenty-two amino acids in protein, fourteen of which can be made by the body, but eight of which must be provided by food. Scientists have found that all eight of the essential amino acids are found in both animal and vegetable foods. For more information on protein, refer to the earlier chapter on this subject.

In the 1980s, there is no longer a concern for protein adequacy on a vegetarian diet. There are no nutrition scientists still concerned about this subject. In fact, nutritionists are unconcerned about any possibility of deficiency except in the

« « « ◯ » » »

case of one nutrient: vitamin B12.

Vitamin B12 is needed for formal functioning of the nervous system. A deficiency causes a sensation of pins-and-needles in the forearms, hands, legs, and feet, leading to weakness, stiffness, unsteadiness, and fatigue. If a person is also deficient in another vitamin named folic acid, then anemia will occur with a B12 deficiency.

When foods are analyzed, vitamin B12 is not found in fruits, vegetables, grains (bread, rice, etc.), or beans. It is only found in meats, dairy products, and eggs. Therefore most nutritionists state that a strict vegan diet will lead to a vitamin B12 deficiency.

Vitamin B12 is exclusively manufactured by bacteria. These bacteria live in a cow's stomach. When they produce B12, it is absorbed into the bloodstream and then ends up in the muscle. When the cow is processed into steak and hamburgers, B12 is found in the meat.

Despite the fact that there is no B12 in non-animal foods, many studies on strict vegetarians have failed to find signs of B12 deficiency. Nonetheless, since scientists have not been able to find B12 in non-animal foods, vegans have been advised to take B12 supplements.

The solution to this mystery has recently been found. For years, it was thought that B12 produced by the bacteria that commonly live in the human intestine could not be absorbed by the body. However, in 1980 a study was published in a major British medical journal which found otherwise. Significant amounts of B12 are produced by intestinal bacteria in an area of the intestine where it can be absorbed. This is probably the reason that strict vegetarians almost never develop a B12 deficiency.

Regardless of diet, a B12 deficiency can occur as a result of sickness in the stomach, intestines, liver, kidneys, or certain other organs. If a person on any type of diet becomes ill, he should be examined by a doctor. A simple blood test can determine if there is a B12 deficiency.

Should all people become vegetarians? I say yes, but this is a matter of individual choice. All people do need to eat minimal

« « « ◯ » » »

amounts of high fat foods, most of which are animal foods. But If animal foods must be used, it is better to eat fish and chicken rather than red meat since the fat content is lower. Also, lowfat dairy products are superior to regular milk and cheese.

But whether the high fat food is cheese, chicken, eggs, nuts, or seeds, it is important to restrict the amount to about 3 ounces per day (1/5 pound).

Is it safe to be a strict vegetarian? Yes. A study of all nutrients including protein and B12, and a thorough examination of all aspects of health, reveals that strict vegetarians are healthier than non-vegetarians.

In fact, if you choose a vegetarian diet, you can expect a general improvement in health. The supposed dangers of vegetarianism are non-existent.

« « « ○ » » »

VITAMINS & MINERALS

Vitamins and minerals are required by the body for normal functioning. A deficiency of vitamin C, iron, or of any other vitamin or mineral can lead to severe illness. It is important to be sure that you are getting enough of these nutrients every day.

Because vitamins and minerals are so important, most people are very concerned about getting enough. Millions of people take food supplements on a daily basis just to be safe. At the first sign of illness, many people will resort to the jar of vitamins. In any discussion of nutrition, it is crucial to cover the subject of vitamins and minerals.

How should we approach this subject? There are thousands of books which will tell you the vitamins and minerals you need, the amounts required, the sources in food for these nutrients, and the diseases which will develop if there is a deficiency. This is common knowledge so there is no need to discuss all of these subjects here.

But it is rare to find answers to our practical questions. What do we have to do on a daily basis to be sure that we are getting enough vitamins and minerals? Do we need to take food supplements? Can we get enough vitamins and minerals from food? How careful must we be when we choose our foods in order to avoid deficiencies? Does modern agriculture produce foods which look good but are deficient in vitamins and minerals? When we are sick, should we take large doses of vitamins, or could this be harmful? These are the significant questions that need to be answered.

One of the most important questions is: do foods grown with today's agricultural methods contain sufficient amounts of vitamins and minerals to provide for our needs?

In the last fifty years, thousands of scientific studies have

« « « O » » »

examined these questions and provided answers. Are foods deficient in vitamins because the soil they were grown in was deficient in vitamins? The answer is no since plants do not get vitamins from the soil. Plants produce these nutrients from carbon dioxide, water, and the energy in sunlight. The plants must produce vitamins for their own needs. The vitamin level in plants is affected only by the weather and amount of sunlight, not the soil.

In one study scientists experimented with tomatoes. A few dozen tomato seeds of identical type were used. Seeds were grown in five widely separated locations in the United States using local soil. At the end of the growing season the tomatoes from all locations were analyzed for vitamin C content. Vitamin C levels varied based on where the tomatoes were grown.

The next year scientists had the soil from these five locations shipped to their laboratory and put in separate containers. The same tomato seeds were grown in the different soils in the same location. When the tomatoes were harvested they were analyzed for vitamin C content. There was no difference found even though different soils were used.

Many similar experiments have convinced scientists that vitamin content will be the same regardless of soil factors. Sunlight and other environmental factors are responsible for the minor differences that are sometimes found. Therefore, if the plant grows, you can be sure that it will provide you with the normal amount of vitamins.

With minerals there is also little reason for concern. Almost all minerals, such as calcium, iron, magnesium, zinc, copper, manganese, boron, and others are needed for normal plant growth. Any textbook on plant nutrition will show how plants use these minerals. Calcium, for instance, is needed to build cell walls in plants. If the soil is too deficient in calcium, the plant will not grow.

If the soil is deficient in a mineral, a plant will not grow properly and the farmer will not be happy. Therefore the soil will be analyzed to see what is lacking. Such soil analysis has been in use for most of this century. If a deficiency is found, the farmer

« « « 〇 » » »

will add the needed mineral to the soil. This is an inexpensive and simple process. Once the mineral has been added, the plant will use it and grow normally. At harvest a food with normal mineral content will be sent to the market.

The only complication comes with the minerals which human beings need but plants do not. There are four such minerals: iodine, chromium, selenium, and cobalt. If all our foods were grown in soil deficient in these minerals, we would have a problem. The plants would grow normally but we would become ill from mineral deficiencies.

Fortunately, however, our food is grown in many areas. On some farms the soil is deficient in iodine, chromium, selenium, or cobalt. But many farms have plenty of these minerals in the soil. A small amount of our food may be low in one of these minerals but most of the food we eat will contain adequate amounts. This protects us from deficiencies.

Since people have begun eating foods grown on a wide variety of soils, there have been no cases of vitamin or mineral deficiencies resulting from a soil deficiency. Deficiencies in human beings have been found but only from poor choices of food, including the use of processed foods which have had their vitamins and minerals destroyed or removed.

Many foods are harvested when they are not yet ripe. Tomatoes, for instance, are picked green so that they can be shipped. Is there a loss of nutrients when a food is harvested before it is ripe? Studies have found that "ripening on the vine or plant does not always produce higher vitamin content." Pineapples ripened on the plant have less vitamin C than those picked green. Tomatoes, however, lose about 30% of their vitamin C when they are picked green. Vitamin content, then, is increased in some foods when picked green, but decreased in others. Since the change in vitamin content is not great either way, we do not need to worry about developing a deficiency as a result of the timing of the harvest.

So now we know that the foods harvested from farms have all the vitamins and minerals we need for optimal health. But what happens after the harvest? Is there a loss of nutrients from the

« « « ◯ » » »

time spent in transport or in storage?

In studies scientists usually measure vitamin C levels since this vitamin is considered to be an overall indicator of nutrient retention after harvest. Many studies have shown that if the food is properly handled after the harvest, there will not be a significant loss of vitamins. Food must not be bruised, dried out, or exposed to warm temperatures. If the food does not look wilted or damaged in the store, if it appears fresh and crisp, you can be sure that most of the vitamins are still intact.

Ensuring optimal vitamin and mineral nutrition with food is easy. In a later chapter I will describe sample dietary plans and show how good nutrition can be easily assured. Generally you must first be sure to eat plenty of raw foods, since cooking destroys a significant amount of vitamins. Also, avoid refined foods such as white flour and white sugar since they have 85% less nutrients than their unrefined counterparts.

If you eat two or three whole fruits, one large raw vegetable salad a day, and avoid white flour and sugar, you will never develop a dietary deficiency of vitamins and minerals. The details of a complete health diet will follow in a later chapter.

« « « O » » »

TO SUPPLEMENT
OR NOT

In the previous chapter, we established that the food we buy in supermarkets, if not refined or overcooked, is actually rich in the vitamins and minerals we need. Some people feel, however, that they should take a supplement just to be safe. Others feel that they should take very large doses of vitamins and minerals to either prevent or treat disease.

In a later chapter, I will describe in detail the recommended diet. An analysis of this diet will show that it is more than sufficent in all vitamins and minerals.

But what if we don't eat healthfully? What if we regularly eat white bread, candy, and canned vegetables, and almost never eat raw fruits and vegetables? Should we take supplements?

The answer is complicated. It is true that if the diet is deficient in vitamin C, then it will be better to take a vitamin C supplement. But many of the negative aspects of a poor diet result from excesses of fats, proteins, and sugars, and no supplement will protect against this type of damage.

Also, there is no supplement that contains every nutrient we need. For instance, it has been known for over ten years that human beings need silicon, tin, and nickel. These trace minerals are found in food, but there is no supplement that includes them. And what about the substances in food that the body needs but which have not yet been identified? The world of nutritional science is not yet perfect. We can only be completely sure that we are getting all the nutrients we need when we eat a wide variety of natural, unrefined foods.

Some people think they do not need to be concerned about eating properly when supplements are used. The supplement supplied everything necessary, so why not eat donuts for breakfast? But this is a dangerous path to take because no pill can

« « « ◯ » » »

protect against damage from the fried fats in the donut, nor can it supply all the nutrients which are missing in an item made from white flour and white sugar.

We have been discussing low dosage supplements. But what about megadoses? A megadose of a vitamin or mineral is a level of dosage that one could never get from food. For instance, if you ate a large amount of fruits and vegetables, you could get 500 milligrams of vitamin C per day from food. The Recommended Dietary Allowance (RDA) is 60. To treat colds, some people take 10,000–20,000 milligrams of vitamin C per day. This is definitely a megadose.

Many people think that if a small amount of vitamins and minerals is good, twenty times more will be better. But a large enough dose will turn the nutrient into a drug, complete with hazardous side effects.

The science of biochemistry teaches that vitamins and minerals are to the body what spark plugs are to a car. If you wanted better performance out of your six cylinder car, would you try to install ten spark plugs? Of course not, since the need for spark plugs in such a car is limited by the number of cylinders. Adding extra spark plugs would not help the engine.

The same is true with vitamins and minerals. The body needs only a limited amount, so 10–100 times more will not be helpful. Vitamins and minerals consumed in excessive amounts cannot be used nutritionally.

Some people feel much better when they take huge amounts of vitamins and minerals and consider this proof that the megadoses fulfilled a nutritional need. But this is not good reasoning since a sense of feeling better can also result from taking a drug. When one takes aspirin for a headache, the pain will disappear. Does this mean that the body needed aspirin to function normally, and that a headache is a sign of aspirin deficiency? Obviously, the answer is no. But when a large dose of vitamin C decreases the congestion of a cold, people believe that the vitamin corrected a deficiency and so the body healed itself more rapidly. The fact is that vitamin C in large doses works like an antihistamine drug, just like those advertised on TV. The

« « « ◯ » » »

elimination of mucus when one has a cold is desirable, since it reduces the load of waste products and toxins in the bloodstream. Antihistamines, including vitamin C, decrease the amount of mucus eliminated, and should therefore be avoided.

To protect your health, remember that megavitamins may function as drugs, not nutrients. Excessively large doses of vitamins cannot be used as nutrients, any more than your car could use one hundred spark plugs. When one feels better after taking a megadose, the effect is the same as when any drug is taken. Drugs suppress symptoms but do not relieve the cause of the symptom.

Vitamins C, B3 (niacin), and E are three of the most common vitamins used in megadose amounts. C is used for colds, B3 to lower cholesterol levels, and E to improve circulation. There is some limited evidence that each will accomplish the desired result, but the effect is pharmacological, not nutritional.

One way to determine if we are dealing with a drug or a nutrient is to look for side effects. Nutrients are used by the body with no signs of any illnesses developing as a result. Drugs interfere with normal body function and signs of illness commonly result.

Megadoses of vitamin C have been proven to destroy red blood cells; irritate the lining of the intestine; cause kidney stone formation; interfere with the use of iron, copper, vitamin A, and bone minerals; cause infertility and fetal death; cause diabetes; and cause rebound scurvy. Scurvy is the disease that results from a true vitamin C deficiency. If you take large amounts of vitamin C for a long time, your body will begin to consistently eliminate more C every day. If you suddenly decide to stop taking C, you will become deficient because it takes a long period of time for your body to begin to eliminate less C every day.

Megadoses of niacin (B3) cause liver damage, elevated blood sugar and uric acid levels, and abdominal pain.

Megadoses of vitamin E result in more deposits of cholesterol in blood vessels, elevated blood fat levels, abnormal clotting of the blood, faster growth of lung tumors, decreased absorption from the intestine of vitamin A and iron, stomach problems, skin

« « « ◯ » » »

rashes, disturbed thyroid gland function, and damage to muscles.

The many side effects which result from the use of mega-vitamins prove that such large doses have a drug, not nutritional, effect.

When healing is necessary, the body will automatically initiate the mechanisms of healing. To support the healing process, the body requires the amount of vitamins and minerals that is easily available in a wholesome diet. Megadoses of nutrients function like drugs: they only suppress symptoms without really "curing" anything, and they are always accompanied by side effects.

« « « O » » »

CALCIUM and DAIRY PRODUCTS

A great concern about getting enough calcium has developed in recent years. Many people believe that it is easy to become deficient in calcium, and the only way to be safe is to use large amounts of dairy products. What are the facts?

The ultimate authority on nutritional needs in the United States is the National Research Council of the National Academy of Sciences. Every five to ten years, they publish an updated version of the book *Recommended Dietary Allowances*. The most recent edition was printed in 1980, with a full chapter on calcium.

The Recommended Dietary Allowance for adults is 800 milligrams per day. This is the amount found in 3 cups of milk, or in 3 1/2 ounces of cheese, or in 2 1/2 cups of almonds, or in 5 medium stalks of broccoli. Calcium is found in many foods, but more is found in dairy products than elsewhere. Since the need is understood to be 800 mg per day, it would seem that dairy products would be required to meet this need because they are so concentrated in calcium.

But how can it be that adult human beings must use the milk of adult cows to get enough calcium? The adult cow does not drink milk. In fact, no other adult mammal uses dairy products. In the biological kingdom, milk is only provided for infants until they are weaned. And, except for human beings, no other lifeform uses the milk of another species.

Usually the discussion of calcium starts and ends with the figure of 800 mg/day. But, there are many other important matters discussed by the National Research Council. For instance, the figure of 800 mg/day is not considered an absolute requirement, but rather as a "guide for planning food supplies." It is recognized that "children do in fact grow healthy bones and that adults remain in calcium balance despite lower calcium intakes."

《 《 《 ◯ 》 》 》

The World Health Organization is quoted as saying that the need for calcium is "between 400 and 500 mg/day because there appeared to be no evidence of calcium deficiency in countries in which calcium intakes were of this order." Many studies have found that an intake of 200 to 400 mg/day of calcium has never been linked with any disease.

So why is the United States RDA 800 mg/day? Because of the "high levels of proteins and phosphorus provided by the U.S. diet." High protein foods are meats, dairy products, beans, nuts, seeds, and eggs. High phosphorus foods are meats, dairy products, and soda pop. Many studies have shown that when a diet high in protein and/or phosphorus is eaten, the body will lose large amounts of calcium in the urine. Therefore, if one eats less than the usual amount of protein and phosphorus, the need for calcium will be far below 800 mg/day.

Cow's milk is much higher in phosphorus than human milk. Also, it is high in protein. Therefore, the more cow's milk you drink, the more calcium you will need. To protect against a deficiency of calcium, most people use large amounts of a food which contributes to calcium deficiency. This is not very sensible.

Of all foods, dairy products are the most likely to cause allergies. For this reason, the American Academy of Pediatrics has recommended that no infant younger than six months of age be given cow's milk products. Doctors commonly find in practice that patients feel better when they avoid dairy products. Also, dairy foods are very high in fat and calories. The animal fat in dairy products is a major part of the cause of heart attacks, strokes, and cancer of the breast, colon, and prostate.

For all the above-listed reasons, I usually recommend that people eat no dairy products. Human beings only need dairy foods in infancy, and at that time they need human milk, not cow's milk. There is a vast difference between these two types of milk. I will discuss this further in the chapter on feeding children.

The eating plan recommended in this book provides far less protein and phosphorus than the customary U.S. diet. Therefore, the need for calcium is much lower than 800 milligrams per day. When the calcium requirement is lower, it can easily be met

« « « ◯ » » »

without using dairy products.

How can a diet be set up to provide enough calcium without milk and cheese? It is easy. Remember that the cow's milk contains calcium because the cow ate plenty of plant foods. If we bypass the cow and eat as the cow eats, we can assure adequate calcium intake without using milk. Plant foods are superior since they do not supply the large amounts of protein and phosphorus found in milk which increase the need for calcium. Also, plant foods are not as rich in fat as are dairy foods, therefore they do not increase the risk of disease.

The following menu provides all the calcium you need on a diet lower than the average in protein and phosphorus: breakfast of one orange (54 mg calcium), one banana (10 mg), one ounce of nuts (50 mg). Lunch of a salad with one carrot (18 mg), one stalk of celery (16 mg), one half cucumber (17 mg), three large leaves of leaf lettuce (51 mg), and one tomato (24 mg). Also for lunch, one slice of whole wheat bread (25 mg), and one cup of cooked green peas (37 mg). For dinner, a repeat of the lunch salad plus 1/2 cup cooked beans (75 mg), and one medium sized stalk of broccoli (158 mg). Total for the day is 661 milligrams. This amount is scientifically proven to be more than adequate, and no dairy products have been used.

What about osteoporosis? Should excessive amounts of calcium be used to prevent this condition? The National Research Council reviewed hundreds of studies and concluded that "it is impossible to prevent osteoporosis in adult life with dietary calcium alone."

Harrison's *Principles of Internal Medicine* is considered a highly respected text. Based on many studies, the authors state that no difference in calcium intake has ever been found between people who have osteoporosis and others of the same age without this condition. In fact, osteoporosis is not primarily from loss of bone calcium, but rather from loss of the fibers in bone upon which calcium is deposited. This text concludes that osteoporosis seems to be related to a high protein intake and a sedentary lifestyle. In the same way that lack of exercise leads to weaker and smaller muscles, many scientists feel that a sedentary existence may

« « « 〇 » » »

weaken the bones and cause osteoporosis.

From the facts, we know that it is easy to get enough calcium on a low protein diet without using any dairy products. Also, osteoporosis is not directly from a calcium deficiency. Why, then, do most people believe that using too little milk and cheese will cause their bones to turn to dust?

The answer is quite simple: dairy industry propaganda. We are surrounded by advertising for milk and cheese. Grade schools teach that children need milk, and they provide it at lunch. Billboards, TV and radio ads, and pamphlets at supermarkets all cry out at us to drink more milk and eat more cheese. Milk has become as American as apple pie and the flag. But remember the facts about milk, calcium, and osteoporosis and don't succumb to this high pressure advertising campaign. Your health will be better as a result.

« « « ◯ » » »

FEEDING BABIES

All the diet ideas discussed so far are suitable for adults and for children past the age of two or three. But feeding infants requires a different approach. How can you assure safe nutrition for your children?

For the first six months of life nature provides a perfect food: human breast milk. This should be the only food for at least the first four months. For the remainder of the first year of life breast milk should be used to the greatest extent possible. Breast milk is nutritious enough to serve as the only food for the first year.

For many years doctors thought that cow's milk was a good substitute for human milk. But scientific studies have proven otherwise. Human milk has many unique properties.

In contrast to cow's milk, human milk contains a growth factor that helps the intestines mature properly. Normal maturation improves the ability of the intestines to process food. It also helps the intestines block absorption of unwanted substances. This reduces the chance of allergies in later life.

Other factors found only in human milk reduce the risk of infectious diseases. Because of these factors, breast-fed babies have far fewer respiratory and gastrointestinal infections.

The fat in human milk is more completely digested than the fat in cow's milk. This is because human milk contains the enzymes needed to digest fat.

Human milk is higher in cholesterol than is cow's milk. The higher level of cholesterol is thought to stimulate the body's mechanisms for dealing with cholesterol. Therefore in later life a person who was breast-fed will be better able to maintain a lower blood cholesterol level.

Obesity in adults is a serious problem since it contributes to the formation of many diseases such as diabetes and heart disease. Breast-fed infants have a lower risk of becoming obese and developing these diseases in adult life.

Breast milk, but not cow's milk, contains the amino acid

« « « ○ » » »

taurine. This chemical is needed for normal maturation of the nervous system. A deficiency of taurine may lead to a lower IQ in adult life.

It is clear from the above that human breast milk is the ideal food for infants. Therefore, it should be used for at least one year. It is healthful to breast-feed even longer.

Occasionally, circumstances make the use of breast milk impossible. Such is the case with adopted babies. If breast milk cannot be used, the best substitute is soy-based formula. Even though breast milk is the ideal, babies fed soy formula can develop normally and be healthy.

Solid foods can be introduced as early as four months. Each infant is different, so the exact timing can vary. When an infant expresses interest in the food his family is eating, he is usually ready for solid foods.

The first foods should be blended or mashed fruits and vegetables. Unsweetened apple sauce, mashed bananas, blended steamed peas or yams, mashed avocado, blended melons, and other such foods are excellent for a start. It is best to introduce only one new food every three days to monitor for allergies.

After a few weeks on fruits and vegetables, cereals may be introduced. It is best to start with oats, rice, and corn. Wheat and rye should not be used until at least six months of age because they cause more allergy problems. To prepare these cereals, cook whole oatmeal and brown rice, then blend. Or buy puffed brown rice and puffed corn, then blend. Mix with expressed breast milk or fruit juice. Always use a three-to-one ratio of fruits and/or vegetables to cereals.

As the months pass and the infant drinks less breast milk, the need for solid foods will increase. After the age of six months, begin to use high protein foods such as tofu, nuts, nut butters, seeds, seed butters, beans, and split peas. Begin with about three tablespoons per day, and increase to ten per day at three years of age. Many of these foods will require blending in the beginning. Dried fruit spreads are good and can be made by blending dried fruit like peaches with water.

If the family chooses a non-vegetarian diet, small amounts of

« « « O » » »

fish and chicken can be used as high protein foods.

In a strict vegetarian diet which includes no meats, fish, dairy products, or eggs, deficiencies are unlikely. The most common ones are of calories, zinc, and vitamin D. On a diet which is not excessive in protein, calcium needs are easily met (see chapter on calcium). Vitamin B12 is produced by intestinal bacteria, therefore this nutrient is rarely a concern (see chapter on vegetarianism).

The calorie need can be met by eating plenty of fruits, dried fruit spreads, nuts and seeds and their butters, and avocados. Zinc is found in beans, nuts, seeds, and tofu. Vitamin D can be formed by the skin when it is exposed to moderate amounts of sunlight.

It is best to have your baby's diet supervised by a knowledgable doctor. In this way you can be sure that the diet is nutritionally complete.

If symptoms of illness develop in your child at any time, see your doctor. But remember certain general rules: when your child is sick and does not want to eat, don't force him. When illness occurs, it is best to feed a light diet of fruits and vegetables, or to skip a few meals altogether. This type of approach in illness is of great help in cases of recurrent ear infections, asthma, chronic colds, and allergies.

You will notice that cow's milk products have not been recommended for use by infants and children. For a more complete discussion of this matter, refer to the chapter on calcium and dairy products. Since cow's milk has been designed by nature only for baby cows, it is unnecessary and often unhealthful for human beings. Protein and calcium needs can easily be met without it. The only appropriate milk for babies is human milk. After weaning no milk of any type is needed.

After the first year or two of life children begin to develop food desires of their own. These desires may include fast food hamburgers, ice cream, cookies, etc. Should parents prohibit all such foods? Or should the child be allowed to eat whatever he wants?

A careful balance must be achieved. Even though junk foods are unhealthful, strict prohibition may cause a child to rebound in the other direction and eat *only* junk foods when he has more

« « « ◯ » » »

control over his diet. But a diet exclusively of junk foods is obviously unacceptable. A workable compromise is to use sweets and other fun foods only for birthdays and holidays.

Raising children is a joy. When you feed your child healthfully he will develop into a strong and vigorous adult. Following the recommendations in this chapter will get your child off to a good start.

« « « ◯ » » »

HERBS

An herb is any type of vegetative growth. All growing plants, therefore, can be classified as herbs. Some herbs, such as lettuce and celery, are foods. Some herbs, such as sweet basil and summer savory are seasonings. Other herbs, such as ginseng and golden seal, may in fact be medicines.

What is the place in a healthful living program for herbs? Obviously the herbs which can be used as foods should be included in generous amounts. Eat plenty of lettuce, tomatoes, cucumbers, carrots, squash, green beans, peas, and all other herbs which can be used as foods.

The herbs which can be used as seasoning are good foods with an appealing aroma and taste. The list of such herbs includes sweet basil, summer savory, marjoram, thyme, oregano, mint, sage, and others. One of the best ways to make food taste good without using salt is to develop combinations of flavorful herbs to sprinkle on food.

The last major category of herbs is the type used as medicines. Herbs in this category are sometimes recommended as "cures" for arthritis, constipation, or even cancer. Should you include medicinal herbs in your health-building program?

It is best to avoid medicinal herbs. The fact is that medicinal herbs in many cases are identical to drugs.

Can you pull any green plant from the soil and safely eat it? Recently, a passenger on a river trip unknowingly tested this concept. When the boat stopped at a beach along the river the passenger picked a pretty green plant and ate it. Within minutes he was dead. The plant happened to be water hemlock, a deadly poison.

Clearly then all green plants are not safe. Some are fine to use as foods, whereas others are extremely toxic. We must be discriminating about which herbs we eat.

You may not know that many medical drugs have come from herbs. Large pharmaceutical companies send teams of researchers

« « « ◯ » » »

to the far ends of the earth to find out what herbs the "natives" use when they become sick. When the scientists find a popular plant, they bring samples back to the lab, isolate the chemicals within the plant that have drug effects, develop methods of synthesizing these chemicals in the laboratory, and market their new drug.

A few hundred years ago pioneers in North America found Indians using the bark of the willow tree to get rid of headache pain. What could seem more natural than the bark of a tree? Yet the reason the bark helps with headaches is because it contains salicylic acid, the chemical in aspirin. Salicylic acid is a drug whether it is found in willow bark or in aspirin tablets.

The foxglove plant contains digitalis, a powerful and potentially dangerous heart drug. The only difference between taking foxglove and purified digitalis is the concentration of digitalis. The adverse effects of foxglove are the same as for digitalis.

There is a new book, *The Honest Herbal*, published in 1981, which is an excellent reference on herbs. Every statement about herbs is backed up by a reference to a scientific journal.

A list of herbs which are proven to be unsafe includes angelica, apricot pits (laetrile), blue cohosh, broom, calamus, canaigre, chaparral, coltsfoot, comfrey, dong quai, eyebright, liferoot, mistletoe, poke root, sassafras, and wormwood. Don't underestimate the danger of these herbs; sassafras and comfrey, for instance, have been proven to cause cancer.

There are many other herbs that are not definitely known to be dangerous, but their safety is in doubt. The list includes bayberry, betony, black cohosh, devil's claw, ginseng, gotu kola, juniper, licorice, lobelia, mormon tea, muira puama, pollen, propolis, raspberry, tansy, and yohimbe. Ginseng, the most popular of this group of herbs, has been linked to disturbances in blood pressure and mood.

Herbs which are considered safe are alfalfa, aloe, arnica, barberry, boneset, borage, buchu, burdock, calendula, chamomile, yarrow, chickweed, chicory, cucurbita, damiana, dandelion, echinacea, fennel, fenugreek, fo-ti, garlic, gentian, goldenseal,

« « « ○ » » »

hawthorn, hibiscus, horehound, horsetail, hyssop, kelp, linden flowers, lovage, mullein, myrrh, nettle, papaya, passion flower, peppermint, red bush tea, red clover, rose hips, rosemary, St. John's wort, sarsaparilla, savory, saw palmetto, scullcap, senega snakeroot, senna, spirulina, uva ursi, valerian, witch hazel, yellow dock, and yucca.

It is important to understand that some of the herbs which are considered safe, such as goldenseal, still may have drug effects in the body, including side effects. Scientists consider aspirin, tylenol, and motrin safe even though they are drugs with many side effects.

Many people resort to herbs in attempts to correct health problems. When the body is not working properly and we feel ill, the body will actively try to correct the problem. We need to help by removing the cause of illness, for instance, stress, improper foods, lack of rest, etc. Attempting to "cure" the disease with herbs will never help the body to heal faster. A medicinal herb will only cover up the symptoms of disease, much like aspirin masks the cause of headache pain. Since the symptoms of disease are not the disease itself, getting rid of symptoms will not improve health.

Greater health can only come from a deeper commitment to healthful living practices. Don't settle for less than the real thing. Dietary changes, exercise programs, more relaxation, and other beneficial changes will dramatically improve your health.

« « « ◯ » » »

EXERCISE

Regular exercise is required to build and maintain good health. Diet is very important but a good diet without regular exercise will not result in good health.

We tend to think that exercise is only for fun. Certainly the type of exercise we choose must be fun or we will not do it regularly. But exercise does far more than make us happy. It is needed to build good health.

In the early days of man's history, regular and strenuous exercise was commonplace. Primitive man had to cover many miles every day in his search for food. The Hopi Indians are said to have run up to twenty miles each way to tend their gardens every day. Roman soldiers often marched forty miles a day dressed in 100 pounds of armor.

Today, however, such strenuous physical activity is rare. Modern civilization has eliminated the need for it. In fact, in many circles, vigorous exercise is unfashionable. People will cruise parking lots to find the closest space so as to avoid walking an extra 100 feet. We will use electric can openers to avoid the effort of manual openers. The life of luxury often seems to be a life of sedentary activities.

But we pay quite a steep price for a sedentary existence. The body requires regular physical activity to build and maintain health. Exercise is not a luxury. It is an absolute necessity.

This does not mean, however, that everyone must run 10 miles a day. The required amount of exercise to build and maintain health is far less. We can definitely get the exercise we need without working so hard that we feel a sense of intense suffering. Exercise can and must be a joy. If we do not truly enjoy our exercise program, it will not last for long.

Why do we need to exercise? The main reason is to maintain the health of the cardiovascular-pulmonary system. This system is responsible for supplying the most essential nutrient of all to the cells of the body: oxygen. The lungs must move oxygen from the

« « « ◯ » » »

air to the bloodstream. The heart must pump the blood to transport oxygen from the lungs to the cells. The blood vessels must carry the oxygen efficiently. Without exercise these tasks will be done poorly and good health will not be achieved.

Exercise strengthens the body systems which supply blood to the cells. This improves the delivery not only of oxygen but also of all vitamins, minerals, proteins, hormones, and other essential nutrients and chemicals. Exercise also pumps the lymphatic system which drains waste products from cells. There is no other pump to power the lymphatic system.

Exercise also helps in weight control. Regular exercise will speed up the body's metabolic rate and increase the amount of muscle so that more calories will be burned 24 hours a day.

Exercise also stimulates the release of endorphins, natural pain killers, from the brain.

Scientific studies have proven time and again that people who exercise regularly in the proper way have a lower risk of heart disease and strokes. These cardiovascular diseases kill more Americans than any other disease, including cancer. Besides conditioning the heart, lungs, and blood vessels, exercise has a beneficial effect on blood cholesterol levels.

Dr. Kenneth H. Cooper, M.D., has done more to promote the benefits of exercise than any other person in this country. Millions of copies of his book *Aerobics* have been sold. He states that exercise can help patients with asthma, bronchitis, emphysema, tuberculosis, heart disease, strokes, congenital heart defects, high blood pressure, varicose veins, stomach ulcers, diabetes, obesity, back pain, arthritis, glaucoma, depression, and anxiety. Obviously exercise is good for you!

Exercise can build health, but only if it is the correct type of exercise. The most healthful type of exercise is aerobic. This is the type that increases the heart rate and makes you breath harder. There are specific guidelines to follow to assure that your exercise program is of the right type.

Other types of exercise which are not aerobic are aimed at muscle strengthening or stretching, relaxation or recreation. Weightlifting will strengthen muscles; it is fine if one is careful, but

« « « ◯ » » »

it is not essential for good health. Muscle stretching exercises are required both before and after aerobic exercises but by themselves, they will not improve health. Relaxation exercises such as Hatha yoga are quite effective in reducing tension, but useless in promoting good cardiovascular-pulmonary health. Recreational exercises such as golf and bowling are enjoyable but not a substitute for aerobic exercises.

Aerobic exercises include walking, jogging, running, hiking, swimming, bicycling, handball, racquetball, basketball, jumping rope, rowing, dancing, ice or roller skating, tennis, and squash. These exercises, and others that have not been listed here, are aerobic because they can be done continuously and steadily with no interruptions for at least twelve minutes at a time and they are vigorous enough to assure that your heart will beat at the training heart rate for the entire twelve minutes.

How do you compute your training heart rate? Count your resting heart rate in bed in the morning before arising by touching a finger to the thumb side of your wrist or the side of your neck. Count the number of heart beats in six seconds, then multiply by 10.

Next, subtract your age from 220. This gives you your maximum heart rate. The final step is to subtract the resting heart rate from the maximum heart rate, multiply this number by .65, then add the resting heart rate to this figure.

For example, take a 40 year old man with a resting heart rate of 70. 220 minus 40 equals 180. 180 minus 70 equals 110. 110 times .65 equals 71.5. 71.5 plus 70 equals 141.5. Therefore, this man must exercise for twelve minutes with his heart beating at the rate of at least 141.5 beats per minute.

This method is the most accurate way of determining the training heart rate. A simpler but less accurate method is to subtract your age from 220, then multiply by .75. Using this method for the 40 year old man above you get 135, which is close to the result of the more accurrate method, but this does not always occur.

There are a few other rules you need to know to exercise the proper way. First, do a slow version of the exercise you have

« « « ◯ » » »

chosen for three to five minutes to warm up before, and then three to five minutes more to cool down after exercising. Second, stretch the muscles you are using both before and after exercising. Third, exercise a minimum of three to four times every week, preferably not on consecutive days.

Recently reports of occasional deaths from exercise have surfaced. To avoid any risk from exercising, get a complete physical exam within one year before starting an exercise program if you are under 30 years of age. If your age is 30 to 35, get a physical exam and a resting electrocardiogram within six months of beginning your program. If you are over 35, get a physical exam and both a resting and stress electrocardiogram within three months of beginning an exercise program.

A resting electrocardiogram will check your heart while you are lying still. A stress electrocardiogram will check your heart when it is working hard as a result of exercising. The doctor will have you run on a treadmill as he performs this test.

Remember, exercise does not have to be painful. It should be fun. There is no need to overexert. Build up your endurance safely, slowly, and progressively. One of many studies which prove that the necessary amount of exercise can be quite comfortable analyzed the effects of walking. It was found that walking at a rate of three miles per hour for thirty minutes at a time, five days a week, was enough to qualify as aerobic exercise if 6.5 pounds was carried on the back. This speed of walking one mile in twenty minutes is not particularly fast. Six and a half pounds is not very heavy. But this is all the exercise you need to do to fulfill your body's needs.

Exercise is crucial for building and maintaining health. Make it a regular part of your life. The investment of time and energy into exercise will pay off in a better quality of life.

« « « ◯ » » »

STRESS

A book on health would be incomplete without a chapter on stress. This is because excessive stress will cause poor health even if we eat properly and exercise regularly. We must recognize the level of stress in our lives and alter our way of living so that the level is not excessive.

What is stress? It is the response of the body to any demands made on it. The body responds to demands by increasing muscle tension, heart rate, blood pressure, hormonal output, plus other changes. These responses increase the body's ability to either face a specific demand and deal with it or to flee from it.

Many people think that the word "stress" implies that there has been a negative experience such as death, divorce, financial loss, or illness. But a significant amount of stress can also be generated by a positive event such as birth, marriage, a desirable job change, or a large inheritance.

Should we attempt to avoid all stress? No. We require a moderate amount of stress in our lives to serve as a stimulus for constructive activities and positive changes. A complete absence of stress would be overwhelmingly stressful!

Therefore the goal is not to eliminate stress but to keep the level of stress within reasonable limits, neither too high nor too low. Sometimes we can moderate the level of stress by changing jobs, homes, or spouses. But usually such changes are not feasible. In most cases, we must deal with stress by changing ourselves. There are many ways to accomplish this which we will discuss later.

What health problems are influenced by stress? All of them. In my practice I rarely see someone whose health problems are totally from stress. But I have never seen anyone who has so little stress that his problems are not at least partially from stress. Therefore everyone can benefit from an effort to learn how to relax.

In the last twenty years a tremendous amount of research has

« « « ◯ » » »

proven that there is a link between mental stress and physical health problems. The following disorders have been proven to be caused or aggravated by stress: heart disease, stroke, high blood pressure, cancer, rheumatoid arthritis, migraine headaches, and respiratory illnesses. But, because excessive stress will reduce overall body health, we can conclude that every health problem will be worsened by stress.

Never underestimate the effect of the mind on health. If you believe that a pin stuck in the heart of a voodoo doll will damage your heart, you may have a heart attack when the pin is inserted. If you believe that a capsule will have a powerful tranquilizing effect when swallowed, you will feel calm after ingesting the capsule even if it contains only flour. This is called the placebo effect. It is well understood by doctors who use it to mobilize the power of the patient's mind to heal health problems.

How do you know if you are under stress? Look at your life with a magnifying glass. How is your home life? Do you fight too often with your spouse, children, or parents? Are the bills stacking up? Does your home need many repairs which you can't take care of at this time?

How is your life outside your home? Do you enjoy your job, or is it frustrating and unfulfilling? Do you get caught in traffic jams every day? Are you exposed to excessive levels of pollution or noise? Do you have satisfying relationships with friends?

The list of possible causes of stress is almost endless. It includes personal injury or illness, retirement, change in financial status, outstanding personal achievements, vacations, Christmas season, violations of the law, etc. We are all unique so those events which are stressful for us will be somewhat different from the events which are stressful for another person.

How should we deal with stress? First, make an effort to change the circumstances of your life so as to minimize stress. Change jobs, catch up on your bills, take the time to repair your home, solve your health problems, postpone retirement, or take other such actions. But if these changes do not sufficiently reduce your stress level, the only further action you can take is to change yourself.

« « « ◯ » » »

One way to help yourself is to become more flexible about your expectations of the nature of your daily life. It is fine to have a preference for a sunny day, but if your expectation is so rigid that you will be depressed if it rains, you need to make some changes.

Do you believe that you will be happy "tomorrow" when you have more money or possessions? If you do, you are only kidding yourself. The secret to happiness is learning how to be happy right now. Remember that "today" is the "tomorrow" that you hoped for "yesterday." If you can't be happy now, you will never be happy later.

Are you unhappy with who you are? We all have our positive and negative attributes and it is fine to have preferences about how you would like to be. But in the meantime while you are trying to improve yourself, accept yourself for the way you are at this very moment.

There are many specific relaxation techniques that you can use. One involves tensing every part of your body at separate times and then mentally willing the part to relax as you release the muscle tension. Start with your feet, then progress to your legs, thighs, buttocks, stomach, chest, back, neck, shoulders, hands, forearms, arms, neck, and face. Tighten the muscles in each area for ten seconds, then mentally ask each area to relax and let go. This is a highly effective technique.

Breathing exercises also work quite well. Lie on the floor on your back, close your eyes and relax. Inhale as you count to ten, then exhale as you count to ten again. Repeat this process ten times.

Meditation is very effective in reducing stress. It can be done in connection with a religion or spiritual science, but it can also be done with no thought whatsoever of religion. Twice a day sit in a quiet corner of your house where you will not be disturbed by people or sounds. Close your eyes, focus your attention on your forehead (don't strain your eyes looking upward), and repeat a calming word for fifteen minutes. Meditation has been proven to produce relaxation very efficiently.

Visualization is another helpful relaxation technique. Sit in a

« « « O » » »

quiet spot, close your eyes, and imagine that you are in a place that you have found relaxing and enjoyable in the past. Your spot might be a secluded beach by the ocean, the shore of a glistening mountain lake, or your garden on a beautiful fall day. Wherever you have found peace, imagine that you are there again. You will be able to create an atmosphere of calm much like the eye of a hurricane.

Biofeedback requires the use of electronic instruments so it is less convenient and more expensive than the other relaxation techniques mentioned, but it is very effective. Instruments are used to measure your level of stress by checking the degree of muscle tension, the amount of perspiration (which is increased with added stress), the nature of your brain waves, and the speed of your heart rate. You get feedback from the instrument which reveals your level of stress. When the muscle is tense, you may hear a louder sound or see a brighter light. By using various relaxation techniques, you can hear the sound lessen, or see the light dim. With biofeedback it is possible to learn exactly which mental changes will produce relaxation.

Occasionally relaxation techniques will not be sufficient. The cause of stress may be a problem which developed many years ago and cannot be clearly identified now. In such cases, a technique such as meditation would have purely symptomatic effects. The stress will return again and again. If this occurs, it is best to consult a professional counselor.

It is definitely possible for people to reduce stress levels. All that is required is effort. When we take the attitude that we are responsible for our physical and mental health we will begin to take positive actions to improve ourselves. When effort is put into reducing stress and learning how to relax, the frequency and intensity of health problems will decrease, and the quality of life will increase. The time to start is now.

« « « ◯ » » »

CHIROPRACTIC

When you need professional help in your quest for health improvement, the best type of doctor to consult is one who is strongly committed to avoiding the use of drugs and surgery except as a last resort. Because of the nature of their training, medical and osteopathic doctors will usually feel quite comfortable with the use of drugs and surgery. There are M.D.s and D.O.s who are exceptions to this general rule and, if you can find one, you may be in luck. But, for the most part, it is best to consult either chiropractic or naturopathic doctors since they know more about the alternatives to drugs and surgery than most other types of doctors.

As a chiropractic doctor, I have found that many people are surprised to learn about the expertise chiropractors have in the field of overall health since chiropractors are often regarded as "back" doctors and nothing more. But times have changed. Chiropractic education in the 1980s is very sophisticated and this qualifies chiropractors to help with a multitude of health problems. The number of class hours in anatomy, physiology, pathology, and diagnosis are the same for both medical and chiropractic students. The differences between the two fields result from the extra training medical students receive in drugs, surgery, and hospital procedures and the extra emphasis chiropractic students receive in spinal adjustments, exercise, physical therapy, and nutrition.

Chiropractic schools are accredited in the same way that medical schools are accredited. The Council on Medical Education (CME) accredits medical schools, while the Council on Chiropractic Education (CCE) and the Straight Chiropractic Accrediting Associaton (SCASA) accredit chiropractic schools. CME, CCE, and SCASA are all licensed by the U.S. Office of Education.

Following graduation medical doctors (MDs) and chiropractic doctors (DCs) are examined, licensed, and regulated by state

« « « ◯ » » »

agencies. In most states insurance companies must pay equally for medical and chiropractic care.

Despite the myths to the contrary, chiropractors do not claim to "cure" diseases by working on the spine. In fact, chiropractors do not claim to cure anything. They simply state that healing is done by the body itself, and that if healing is possible without the use of drugs and surgery then it will be appropriate for the patient to choose a chiropractor for his doctor. Remember that chiropractors only work with health problems that can be helped without drugs and surgery. They are trained well enough to know when a patient needs medical care, so a referral to a medical doctor is made when necessary.

Modern chiropractors are usually able to provide education regarding diet, exercise, and stress reduction. They can supervise the changes in such lifestyle patterns which may be necessary to allow healing to occur. Chiropractors can also help remove obstacles to healing by using spinal adjustments.

What problems can spinal adjustments help? Most people associate the word "chiropractic" with back problems. This is because chiropractic care is superlative for such problems, of which there is an epidemic. Most people are not happy relying on drugs such as pain killers and muscle relaxers which only cover up the problem. They prefer to get to the root of the difficulty and chiropractic is the most effective measure available.

But many internal health problems will also respond to chiropractic care. The nervous system controls and coordinates all functions in the body. All nerve impulses originate in the brain, flow to the spinal cord, and then to nerves which feed all the organs, glands, muscles, and other tissues of the body. If the spinal nerves are stressed by a problem in the spine, the nerves will not work properly and the organ on the other end of the nerve will not function healthfully.

Chiropractors often care for patients suffering from asthma, bronchitis, colitis, irritable colon, constipation, painful menstrual periods, shingles, high blood pressure, nervousness, chest pain, the common cold, sinusitis, insomnia, gastritis, rapid heart beat, dizziness, and ringing in the ears.

« « « ◯ » » »

Chiropractic is sometimes surrounded by an air of controversy. Both supporters and critics are fervent in their beliefs. It has been difficult to know the facts about chiropractic, at least until 1979 when an independent and unbiased report by a special commission of the New Zealand government was published.

Some of the most important conclusions of this 377 pages report are: "modern chiropractic is a soundly-based and valuable branch of health care in a specialized area neglected by the medical profession . . . worthy of public confidence and support."

"Chiropractors are the only health practitioners who are necessarily equipped by their education and training to carry out spinal manual therapy, which can be effective in relieving musculoskeletal symptoms such as back pain, and other symptoms known to respond to such therapy, such as migraine."

"In a limited number of cases where there are organic and/or visceral symptoms, chiropractic treatment may provide relief. Chiropractors should, in the public interest, be accepted as partners in the general health care system. Much medical criticism of chiropractors is based on simple ignorance."

Remember that these conclusions are not those of a chiropractic or of a medical group. The source is an independent, unbiased government commission. Therefore you can rely on their accuracy. In the bibliography of this chapter you will find the names of books which contain references to scientific studies which echo the findings of the New Zealand commission.

In cases of cancer, tuberculosis, rabies, and other such conditions, medical care will be required. But when drugs and surgery are not needed, as is the case with the vast majority of health problems, it is best to consult a chiropractor or naturopath first.

Chiropractic and naturopathic doctors will often prescribe healthful foods, regular exercise, extra rest, reduced stress, and spinal adjustments. With aches and pains from injuries and accidents, and with some internal conditions, spinal adjustments will usually have a dramatic effect.

Regardless of the type of doctor you see or the nature of the treatment you receive, always remember that it is the "Inner

« « « O » » »

Doctor" that is responsible for healing. If your health problem is relatively minor, you may regain good health simply by following the program outlined in the book. However if the problem is more serious, be sure to get professional help from a licensed doctor.

« « « O » » »

DRINKING WATER

You may be endangering your health if the water you drink comes from your local water system. Cancer-causing chemicals are found in almost every city water supply in this country. The quantity of these chemicals is high enough to cause a significant number of cancer cases throughout the land.

How can this be so? Certainly it is understandable that a city which draws its water from a river polluted by industrial wastes would have contaminated tap water. But what about a city which gets its water from the mountains or from deep wells in the wilderness? Won't this water be pure and safe?

Sadly, the answer is no. And the reason is chlorination, the process which saves us from bacterial contamination. Even the purest water from the wilderness contains bits and pieces of leaves, roots, bark, and other such natural products. The smallest particles cannot be filtered out by any city water system. These small particles of organic material are harmless. But when chlorine is added, as it always is, the chlorine combines with these particles and dangerous cancer-causing chemicals are formed.

Examples of chemicals formed in this manner are chloroform, methylene chloride, and carbon tetrachloride. Many of these chemicals are proven carcinogens. Don't be deluded into a sense of security because of the small amounts of these chemicals present. Scientists strongly feel that ingesting even a small amount of such carcinogens for many years will significantly increase your risk of developing cancer.

In 1985 the International Conference of the Occupational and Environmental Significance of Industrial Carcinogens was held in Bologna, Italy. Scientists from all around the world concluded that "there is no safe threshold of exposure to toxic chemicals—there appears to be no level below which a cancer-causing chemical will not cause cancer." Dr. Arthur Upton, former chief of the National Cancer Institute, stated that "we are faced with the facts that there are an unknown number of chemicals

« « « ◯ » » »

that may cause cancer, and if we don't find them and eliminate them from the environment, we may be exposing future generations to unnecessary risks of cancer."

Even if your tap water tastes and smells good, there may be trouble. Most of the cancer-causing chemicals have no taste or smell.

Besides the hazardous chemicals that are formed when chlorine is added to water, there are other sources of danger. For example, consider what recently happened in Phoenix, Arizona.

In the early 1980s scientists for the first time tested local water supplies for trichloroethylene (TCE), a known carcinogen. They were alarmed to find hazardous levels of this chemical in reservoirs supplying a large section of the city. Measures were immediately taken to eliminate the TCE. Fortunately they were successful.

Then scientists attempted to uncover the source of the TCE. TCE is a solvent which was once commonly used by electronic firms. Around the time of World War II, TCE was dumped onto vacant land in the Phoenix area. This land has in more recent times been developed into residential areas. The TCE remained in the ground and it slowly seeped into the water supply.

This means that for the last forty years people in Phoenix have been drinking water polluted with a known carcinogen, TCE. Nobody knew because tests for TCE had never been performed. Scientists cannot accurately guess at the number of cancer cases which have been partially or completely caused by TCE, but they fear that the number is not small.

Can Phoenix residents now breathe a sigh of relief since TCE has been removed from the water supply? No. Ken Schmidt, a local water-quality consultant, has stated that "it's likely that, in the future, when more expensive and detailed studies can be conducted, pollutants more dangerous than TCE will be found in ground water." David Kreamer, a hydrology professor at Arizona State University, has said that TCE pollution is "just the tip of the iceberg" as the search expands for other toxic chemicals that have seeped into the groundwater. He states that we will find "more chemicals in the course of the discovery process."

« « « ◯ » » »

What about those of you who do not live in Phoenix? Should you rest easy? Not if you are smart. An Environmental Protection Agency report has found 180,000 surface impoundments of dangerous liquid wastes in 80,263 different locations throughout the country which are contaminating local water supplies. The government accounting office found more than 146,000 violations of drinking water regulations by 28,000 of the nation's 65,000 community water systems. In most cases the violations were failure to test drinking water for mercury, lead, pesticides, carcinogenic chemicals formed from the combination of chlorine and natural organic materials, and radioactivity.

Because of the danger from drinking water pollution, U.S. Representative Toby Moffet, Connecticut, stated in 1982 that "ground water contamination is the most serious public health and environmental problem now facing this nation."

It is ironic that water contamination is such a serious health problem when you consider how easy it is to avoid the danger. All you have to do is drink purified water and use tap water only for bathing, laundry and other household need. Inexpensive purified water eliminates the risk to your health from contaminated tap water.

What is the best source of purified water? Should you use filters that attach to your faucet, filters that are spliced into your water line, bottled drinking or spring water, bottled distilled water, or some other alternative?

Studies of home water filters show that they are helpful, but not sufficient. Home water filters, usually made of activated carbon, will improve the taste and smell of water but will not remove all of the cancer-causing chemicals. An EPA study of thirty-one filters of all types found that one removed 87% of a major type of hazardous chemical, another removed 55%, but the other twenty-nine filters removed less than 32% of the chemical. Filters are therefore unreliable.

This leaves bottled water as the best alternative. Should you use spring water or distilled water? Since the purity of bottled spring and drinking water is not always known, the best alternative is distilled water. Distilled water is the purest water on

« « « ◯ » » »

the market and therefore it is the best alternative. You can have five gallon jugs delivered to your home. The average family will use about $20 of water per month. There is no evidence that distilled water will cause mineral deficiences in the body even though it contains no minerals.

The prevalence of drinking water contamination in our country is overwhelming. The danger of the chemicals which contaminate the water is chilling. Don't wait for your local government to do an effective job of purifying your water supply. The technology to do this is not available and it may be prohibitively expensive when it is. But you can start protecting yourself today by drinking only pure bottled distilled water.

« « « ◯ » » »

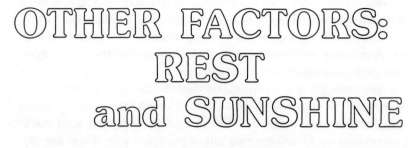

OTHER FACTORS: REST and SUNSHINE

One of the most crucial needs of the body is for sufficient rest and sleep. Yet this need is commonly neglected in so-called "modern" civilization. Many people feel that they should be on the go every minute and that time spent sleeping is wasted because it is unproductive. This attitude is a major cause of poor health.

Many years ago the need for sufficient rest was well understood. One doctor said that "the rest-cure is the only scientific form of cure known to our day." In previous chapters we have established that healing is exclusively done by the body itself. In order to heal, the body must have the energy required to fuel the activities of healing. If the body is exhausted sufficient rest will be required to restore the necessary powers of healing through the process of recuperation.

The need for rest is undeniable and logical. We all have been taught the importance of plenty of rest in maintaining and restoring good health. Yet in actual daily practice the vast majority of people devote far too little time to rest and sleep.

Sufficient rest is required to stay healthy. During those periods of time when one feels an overall sense of vigor and good health, all that is usually needed is a good night's sleep. How much sleep is needed? This varies since one person may be sufficiently rested with six hours of sleep each night while another may need ten hours. The only way to know how much sleep you need is to take an honest look at yourself.

Do you arise in the morning bright-eyed, refreshed, and energetic? Or do you drag yourself out of bed and only wake up after your system has been whipped with three cups of coffee? If

« « « ◯ » » »

you fall into the latter category, you are making daily withdrawals from your "savings account" of energy reserves. Physical "bankruptcy" in the form of illness will inevitably result.

When you feel exhausted at night, do you force yourself to stay awake to finish that one last report, clean out that one final drawer, or finish that one last chapter? If this is your regular style, watch out. A physical collapse is in the making.

If you are not in good health, if you feel tired all the time and "come down" with every bug you are exposed to, if you feel too exhausted to exercise, then more radical recuperative measures may be necessary. You may need a period of physicial rest much longer than a good night's sleep. Two or three or more days in bed may be needed.

Besides physical rest of your muscles, you may need physical rest of your internal organs. Fasting is the finest method for achieving complete internal rest. When the organs of the body are given a respite from digestion, absorption, and elimination of food and its byproducts, a profoundly deep type of rest occurs. This type of rest will give the body a chance to recuperate the energy it needs to heal itself. Safe and successful fasts do, of course, require the supervision of a doctor experienced in fasting.

Sometimes muscle and organ rest is not enough. In such cases, mental rest will be needed. Some people with serious health problems will go to bed and rest their muscles and go without food to rest their organs. But while in bed they will attempt to read five books a day, or finish their PhD dissertation, or buy and sell stocks on the phone, or some other mentally exhausting activity. But since mental exhaustion produces as much fatigue as eating large amounts of food or running many miles, physical recuperation and reinvigoration will not occur. Sometimes it is necessary to force ourselves to slow our thinking processes from a gallop to a crawl.

Never underestimate the potent effect that physical and mental exhaustion will have on your health. And never forget the dramatic effect that sufficient rest will have in rebuilding health. Take an honest look at your life and see if you are sowing seeds of health or disease with the level of rest which you permit yourself

« « « O » » »

every day.

How does natural sunlight fit into the scheme of health-building? Sufficient exposure to the sun is as important as proper food, exercise and all the other lifestyle measures that influence health status.

One of the first promoters of sunlight as a heath-building measure was Arnold Rickli of Switzerland in the 1800s. He stated that: "Man is made to live in the open air; therefore, when exposed to the action of light, air, and sun, he is in his real element. As a natural agent, water takes only an inferior place, above it comes air, while light takes precedence over every other natural agent, and is the greatest essential wherever organic life exists. The nervous system, which is an inherent principle of our organism, is acted upon by light, especially through the skin."

For many years scientists were skeptical about the need for sunlight, but recent research has confirmed that the early teachings of Rickli were correct. A scientific conference on sunlight, sponsored by the New York Academy of Sciences in 1984, revealed many dramatic effects of sunlight.

The most well known effect of skin exposure to sunlight is the production of vitamin D by the skin. This vitamin is needed for the body to absorb dietary calcium. Some scientists think that bone loss in the elderly may be partly related to a vitamin D deficiency from lack of exposure to sufficient sunlight.

Even more fascinating is the discovery that when the eyes are exposed to sunlight they send a message to the pineal gland in the brain which stops the secretion of the hormone melatonin by this gland. In this way, sunlight results in many dramatic changes in body functioning.

The effect on melatonin secretion, or some other mechanism that is not yet understood, is thought to be a factor in depression, decreased alertness, increased sleepiness, and decreased sexual activity which people experience in the winter when there is far less natural light. One psychiatrist found that exposing patients to ultrabright lights relieved symptoms of depression faster than any known anti-depressant drug.

We can conclude, therefore, that sufficient sunlight is

« « « ◯ » » »

required just as much as sufficient food and oxygen. To maintain or restore health, sunbaths are required. How much time should you spend in the sun? In the summer don't go out in the middle of the day. Rather, spend a half-hour in mid-morning or mid-afternoon in the sun. Don't allow yourself to be overheated since this is extremely fatiguing.

During the other seasons of the year expose your skin to the sun during mid-day. The sun will not be strong enough then to harm you in any way.

As with any other need of the body, such as for vitamins and water, you can harm yourself with too much sun. Excessive sunbathing will prematurely age the skin and sometimes even cause skin cancer. The goal of sunbathing to build health does not require the amount of time needed to develop a deep brown tan. Nor should you ever allow your skin to burn from sunlight exposure. Be moderate and careful when you sunbathe and no harm will result.

The proper amount of sunbathing will improve your health, as revealed by the recent conference on sunlight and health. Even though many benefits of sunlight are known, one researcher at the conference was quoted as saying that "the best is yet to come." But don't wait for science to spell out every detail. Make regular sunbathing a part of your life and enjoy the health benefits now.

« « « 〇 » » »

DIET and MENU PLANS

Following are examples and comparisons of different recommended diet plans. The diets described are the standard United States Dietary Allowances (USDA) plan, our Health-Building Diet, and a Vegan Diet at three different caloric levels. The purpose of the comparisons is to show that it is quite easy to fulfill all nutritional needs without following the government's four food group plan; moreover, *the alternative plans described are far more healthful.*

The USDA diet claims that it is necessary on a daily basis to use foods from each of its four groups of foods: "1. Drink two or more cups of milk. 2. Eat two or more servings of meat. 3. Use four or more servings of fruits and vegetables. 4. Eat four or more servings of whole grain or enriched grain products (whole wheat or white bread, for example)."

The "Health-Building Diet," as you will see through the comparisons, is far more healthful than the USDA Diet. The Health-Building Diet described below contains no meat, dairy products, or eggs. However if you do not choose to be a vegetarian, you can substitute small amounts of chicken and/or fish for the seeds, nuts, and dairy products listed.

The USDA diet is 49% fat whereas the Health-Building diet is 26% fat. Scientists have proven that a high fat diet causes heart disease, strokes, and many types of cancer (see chapters on these subjects). The average American consumes a 40% fat diet. The American Heart Association, National Cancer Institute, and other authorities have recommended that the percent of fat be reduced at least to 30%, and down to 20% in high risk cases (diabetics, heart patients, etc.). The USDA diet provides a dangerously high amount of fat of the worst kind: saturated fat with cholesterol. The Health-Building diet contains a safe amount of fat, with no

« « « ◯ » » »

saturated fat or cholesterol.

The USDA diet is deficient in vitamins B1, B2, B3, and fiber. The Health-Building diet provides plenty of all the vitamins and minerals. There is more than enough calcium and protein, despite the lack of meat and dairy products.

The comparison between these two diets should forever put to rest the contention that the USDA Four Food Group plan is the only way to secure adequate nutrition. In fact, the following charts prove that the USDA plan is inferior to many other food plans, including the Health-Building diet described here.

Following the Health-Building diet is a food plan containing no concentrated protein foods, such as animal products or nuts and legumes. It will demonstrate that well-balanced nutrition can be obtained without the use of high protein foods; that more than adequate protein can be supplied through eating vegetables, fruits, and grains.

Typical USDA Four Food Group Diet

Meat Group: 4 ounces beef steak, grilled; 2 ounces bacon, fried; 1 egg, fried

Milk Group: 2 cups pasteurized milk

Fruit and Vegetable Group: 1 medium carrot, 1 medium orange, 1 potato, small lettuce and tomato salad

Bread and Cereal Group: 3 slices white enriched bread; 1 serving cornflakes

Miscellaneous Additions: 5 ounces sugar, 2 tablespoons butter, 2 tablespoons margarine, 1 tablespoon mayonnaise

« « « ◯ » » »

The Health-Building Diet

Breakfast: 1 large peach (200 grams), 1 large apple (200 grams), 2 pears (400 grams)

Lunch: Romaine lettuce (8 leaves), young and tender collards (4 small leaves), celery (2 cups diced), 2 medium-sized tomatos, alfalfa sprouts (1 cup), almonds (1/2 cup), sunflower seeds (1/3 cup).

Dinner: Romaine lettuce (8 leaves), 1 cucumber, mung bean sprouts (1 cup), parsley (2/3 cup chopped), broccoli (1 small stalk), 2 large baked yams

Diet Comparison Chart

	Health-Building Diet	USDA Diet	R.D.A. Standard
Calories	2266	2692	2800
Protein	69 grams	78 grams	55 grams
Fat	65 grams	146 grams	
Calcium	1531 mg	829 mg	800 mg
Phosphorus	1531 mg	1265 mg	800 mg
Sodium	503 mg	2781 mg	300 mg (approx.)
Potassium	8819 mg	2967 mg	2000 mg (approx.)
Vitamin A	37,911 IU	8427 IU	5000 IU
Vitamin B1	2.83 mg	1.14 mg	1.4 mg
Vitamin B2	2.87 mg	1.50 mg	1.70 mg
Vitamin B3	24 mg	11 mg	18 mg
Vitamin C	727 mg	140 mg	60 mg
Fiber	30 grams	2.4 grams	10 grams (approx.)

1921 Calorie Vegan Health-Building Diet

The following is a nutritional breakdown of a 1921 calorie vegan diet compared to the RDA standards for a female 30–51 years of age.

Breakfast: Melon (2 wedges watermelon, 1/2 cantalope, 1/2 honeydew, 1814 grams total)

Lunch: Lettuce (170 grams, about 7 leaves), alfalfa sprouts (100 grams), banana (357 grams), and grapes (226 grams, about 1 1/2 cups)

Dinner: Large Salad (repeat of previous page's lunch), steamed vegetables (broccoli, cauliflower, collards, 900 grams or 6 cups total); and baked potato (312 grams) with avocado (54 grams, about 1/5 of an avocado)

Nutrient Values (%RDA)

KCalories	2639 Kc	(98%)	Carbohydrate	559.4 Gm	(0 %)
Protein	73.55 Gm	(131%)	Tryptophan	870.1 Mg	(414%)
Threonine	2575 Mg	(461%)	Isoleucine	3046 Mg	(363%)
Leucine	4725 Mg	(423%)	Lysine	3446 Mg	(411%)
Methionine	1038 Mg	(298%)	Cystine	783.2 Mg	(224%)
Phenyl-anine	2953 Mg	(528%)	Tyrosine	1540 Mg	(275%)
Valine	3927 Mg	(402%)	Fat	30.25 Gm	(0 %)
Fiber–Crude	23.39 Gm	(0 %)	Fiber–Diet	95.09 Gm	(0 %)
Cholesterol	0.000 Mg	(0 %)	Potassium	8639 Mg	(230%)
Magnesium	827.5 Mg	(236%)	Iron	23.92 Mg	(239%)
Vitamin A	46498 IU	(930%)	Thiamin	3.016 Mg	(215%)
Riboflavin	2.486 Mg	(155%)	Niacin	29.74 Mg	(165%)
Vitamin B6	6.016 Mg	(273%)	Folacin	930.1 Mg	(233%)
Panto-acid	8.660 Mg	(157%)	Calcium	1125 Mg	(141%)
Phosphorus	1334 Mg	(167%)	Vitamin C	776.9 Mg	(1295%)
Alcohol	0.000 Gm	(0 %)	Copper	3.394 Mg	(136%)
Manganese	7.305 Mg	(195%)	Vitamin E	19.76 Mg	(198%)
Sugar	178.1 Gm	(0 %)	Chromium	0.279 Mg	(223%)
Selenium	0.242 Mg	(194%)	Caffeine	0.000 Mg	(0 %)

Protein: 10%   Carbohydrate: 80%   Fat: 10%   Alcohol: 0%

2070 Calorie Vegan Health-Building Diet

The following is a nutritional breakdown of a 2070 calorie vegan diet compared to the RDA standards for a male over 51 years of age.

Breakfast: 1 grapefruit (246 grams), 3 oranges (524 grams), pumpkin seeds (56 grams-about 1/3 cup)

Lunch: Large salad (lettuce, cabbage, alfalfa sprouts, sweet pepper, tomato, 680 grams total); and 2 baked potatoes (312 grams)

Dinner: Large Salad (repeat of lunch), steamed vegetables (broccoli, cauliflower, collards, 900 grams or 6 cups total); and brown rice (487 grams, about 2 cups cooked)

Nutrient Values (%RDA)

KCalories	2070 Kc	(86%)	Fat	36.00 Gm	(0 %)
Cholesterol	0.000 Mg	(0 %)	Carbohydrate	397.0 Gm	(0 %)
Protein	76.80 Gm	(137%)	Threonine	2588 Mg	(463%)
Isoleucine	3192 Mg	(381%)	Leucine	4702 Mg	(421%)
Lysine	4072 Mg	(486%)	Methionine	1127 Mg	(323%)
Cystine	622.0 Mg	(178%)	Phenyl-Anine	2828 Mg	(506%)
Tyrosine	1613 Mg	(289%)	Valine	4195 Mg	(429%)
Thiamin	2.925 Mg	(244%)	Riboflavin	2.592 Mg	(185%)
Niacin	27.00 Mg.	(169%)	Vitamin B6	4.030 Mg	(183%)
Folacin	1248 Ug	(312%)	Panto-Acid	8.486 Mg	(154%)
Vitamin A	87080 IU	(1742%)	Vitamin C	1263 Mg	(2105%)
Vitamin E	15.50 Mg	(155%)	Vitamin K	1732 Ug	(1650%)
Calcium	1488 Mg	(186%)	Chromium	0.359 Mg	(287%)
Copper	3.436 Mg	(137%)	Iron	30.40 Mg	(304%)
Magnesium	972.0 Mg	(278%)	Manganese	4.321 Mg	(115%)
Phosphorus	1661 Mg	(208%)	Potassium	8156 Mg	(217%)
Selenium	0.215 Mg	(172%)	Zinc	15.00 Mg	(100%)
Fiber-Crude	24.70 Gm	(0 %)	Fiber-Diet	89.20 Gm	(0 %)
Alcohol	0.000 Gm	(0 %)	Ash	25.30 Gm	(0 %)
Sugar	126.0 Gm	(0 %)			

Protein: 14%   **Carbohydrate: 72%**   **Fat: 15%**   **Alcohol: 0%**

2639 Calorie Vegan Health-Building Diet

The following is a nutritional breakdown of a 2639 calorie vegan diet compared to the RDA standards for a male 30–51 years of age.

Breakfast: Oatmeal (468 grams, about 2 cups cooked); raisins (27 grams, about 1/6 cup); apple (138 grams); banana (342 grams)

Lunch: Large salad (repeat of previous 680 gram salad); baked potato (468 grams); avocado (86 grams, about 1/3)

Dinner: Steamed vegetables (broccoli, cauliflower, collards, 900 grams or 6 cups total); brown rice (585 grams, about 2 cups cooked); dates (75 grams, about 1/2 cup)

Nutrient Values (%RDA)

KCalories	1921 Kc	(96%)	Protein	60.90 Gm	(138%)
Carbohydrate	427.0 Gm	(0 %)	Tryptophan	521.0 Mg	(320%)
Threonine	1936 Mg	(445%)	Isoleucine	2086 Mg	(319%)
Leucine	2891 Mg	(332%)	Lysine	3100 Mg	(475%)
Methionine	609.0 Mg	(224%)	Cystine	459.0 Mg	(169%)
Phenyl-Anine	1565 Mg	(360%)	Tyrosine	1121 Mg	(258%)
Valine	2389 Mg	(314%)	Fat	23.20 Gm	(0 %)
Fiber-Crude	30.30 Gm	(0 %)	Fiber-Diet	74.20 Gm	(0 %)
Cholesterol	0.000 Mg	(0 %)	Potassium	10783 Mg	(288%)
Magnesium	865.0 Mg	(288%)	Iron	22.50 Mg	(125%)
Phosphorus	1149 Mg	(144%)	Calcium	1336 Mg	(167%)
Copper	3.396 Mg	(136%)	Manganese	6.414 Mg	(171%)
Vitamin A	69101 IU	(1728%)	Thiamin	3.176 Mg	(318%)
Riboflavin	2.857 Mg	(238%)	Niacin	25.20 Mg	(194%)
Vitamin B6	7.751 Mg	(388%)	Folacin	1270 Ug	(318%)
Vitamin B12	0.000 Ug	(0 %)	Panto-Acid	11.00 Mg	(200%)
Vitamin C	1179 Mg	(1965%)	Vitamin E	9.866 Mg	(123%)
Vitamin K	1503 Ug	(1431%)	Alcohol	0.000 Gm	(0 %)
Ash	29.40 Gm	(0 %)	Sugar	294.0 Gm	(0 %)
Chromium	0.257 Mg	(206%)	Caffeine	0.000 Mg	(0 %)

Protein: 11%   Carbohydrate: 79%   Fat: 10%   Alcohol: 0%

No Concentrated Protein Food Plan

The following food plan includes no animal products or concentrated sources of proteins such as nuts. Its purpose is to demonstrate that a well-balanced and nutritious diet can be composed without the use of animal products or nuts. The nutritive values can be found in the *USDA Handbook #456.*

Breakfast: Orange juice (8 ounces), strawberries (1 cup), banana (one large), papaya (1 half), lettuce (4 leaves), celery (3 stalks).

Lunch: Mixed vegetable salad containing lettuce (4 leaves), carrot (one large), cabbage (one cup), sweet red pepper (one small), tomato (one medium), celery (one stalk), lemon (1/4 wedge). Also: avocado (1 half) and potato (one large baked).

Dinner: Mixed vegetable salad (same as lunch), steamed cauliflower (one cup), broccoli (1 stalk), kale (one cup), brown rice (one cup dry, approximately 3 cups cooked)

2000 Calorie No Concentrated Protein Food Plan
Compared With
RDA Standards for a 23–50 Year Old Female

	Rational Diet	R.D.A. Standard	Percentage Difference
Calories	2000	1600–2400	
Protein	59.4 grams	44 grams	+35%
Calcium	1114 mg	800 mg	+39%
Phosphorus	1393 mg	800 mg	+74%
Iron	21.8 mg	10 mg	+118%
Sodium	542 mg	less than 3300 mg	
Potassium	7869 mg	5625 mg	+40%
A, carotene	60,690 IU	5000 IU	+1114%
B-1, thiamine	2.55 mg	1.4 mg	+82%
B-2, riboflavin	2.19 mg	1.6 mg	+37%
B-3, niacin	28.7 mg	18 mg	+59%
C, ascorbic acid	1485 mg	60 mg	+2375%

CONCLUSION

In writing a conclusion for this book, I tried to center on the most important overall theme that I have presented. In a nutshell, here it is: *You* make the choices that will determine whether or not you are in good health and, with the tools you have now learned, *you can unleash your inner doctor and achieve superlative health.*

So-called "common sense" today holds that your health is not subject to your control. Rather you are completely at the mercy of whatever pollen or virus or bacteria that floats your way. This philosophy maintains that the causes of most illnesses, from the common cold to cancer, are unknown and that you are powerless to avoid them.

But nothing could be further from the truth! Whether or not you are in good health depends upon the choices you make every day. If you choose to be in good health, you will not be affected by the pollen, viruses, and bacteria to which you are exposed. You will rarely develop a cold and, if you do, you will know exactly what you did to cause it. Your risk of cancer will be reduced by over 90%.

Besides being realistic and scientific, this philosophy of health is delightfully liberating. When one has been sick for many years, has become completely "sick of being sick," yet can only find answers such as "we don't know why this problem has developed," or "maybe it's all in your head and you need to see a psychiatrist," a sense of devastating depression and hopelessness will result.

However when you understand that *you* can dramatically improve your health status by making changes in lifestyle, you will become flooded with a sense of power. And the better you feel as a result of the new choices you make, the greater will be your sense of power in life. Eventually you will become fully "empowered" as the truth fully dawns: *control of your health destiny lies completely in your own hands.* What a sense of freedom this brings!

« « « ◯ » » »

So let the end of this book be a true beginning for you. Go on from here and use the tools you have learned and the recipes that follow to dramatically improve your health. This process has been, is now, and will in the future manifest itself in the lives of scores of people. I hope that you are the next.

My Very Best Regards,

Alan M. Immerman, D.C.
Chiropractic Physician
Professional Natural Hygienist

« « « ◯ » » »

RECIPE BOOKS and RECIPES

There are many books on the market which contain recipes which are consistent with the dietary principles presented in this book. The following information will introduce you to these recipe books and tell you briefly how to use them.

The first is *The McDougall Plan Recipes, Volumes One and Two.* All the recipes in this book are vegetarian with no meat, eggs, or dairy products. No oil is used which makes this book even more attractive than most. For the average person who is not suffering from a serious health problem, the cooked food recipes in this book can be used for 1/4 to 1/3 of the diet. Eat raw fruits and vegetables for the remainder of the diet. This book can be purchased from Dr. John McDougall, St. Helena Hospital, Deer Park, California 94576.

The second recipe book is *The Uncook Book: Raw Food Adventures to a New Health,* by Elizabeth and Dr. Elton Baker. This book can be purchased from Communication Creativity, 433 Fourth St., P.O. Box 213, Saguache, CO 81149. It is an excellent introduction to the world of raw food diets. There is excessive concern, however, with the importance of food combining. Also, honey is recommended even though it is only slightly less destructive than white sugar. Avoid the vinegar in the recipes since it tends to make the blood too acidic. Also, be cautious in the use of spices since some can be irritating to the body.

The third book is *Live Foods–Nature's Perfect System of Human Nutrition,* by George and Doris Fathman. It is available from the Ehret Publishing Co., P.O. Box 338, Beaumont, CA 92223. It is best to minimize the use of certain foods recommended in this book such as honey, gelatin, and vegetable oil. Otherwise this is a good recipe book.

The fourth book is *Light Eating for Survival,* by Marcia Madhuri

« « « ◯ » » »

Acciardo, available from 21st Century Publications, P.O. Box 702, Fairfield, IA 52556. Again, avoid the honey, oil, and harsh spices found in the recipes.

The fifth book is *The Vegan Kitchen*, by Freya Dinshah, available from the American Vegan Society, 501 Old Harding Highway, Malaga, NJ 08328. The main food found in this book which you should avoid is oil.

The sixth book is *Ten Talents*, by Frank J. Hurd, D.C., and Rosalie Hurd, B.S., available from the authors at Box 86A–Route 1, Chisholm, MN 55719. Some of the recipes include milk and eggs which should be used in extreme moderation or completely avoided. Also, minimize the use of honey, baking powder, and oil.

The seventh book is *Recipes for Longer Life*, by Ann Wigmore, available from the Avery Publishing Group, Inc., Wayne, NJ. Avoid the honey, oil, and molasses used in many of the recipes. Also, don't use the fermented foods recommended in this book. Fermenting food causes a deterioration in the food which is much the same as the rotting process. Food is not made healthier by letting it sit out at room temperature while bacteria decompose it. Also, there is no miraculous healing power to wheat grass juice which is recommended in this book. Eat a few leaves of green lettuce and you will get as much benefit as you would from drinking wheat grass juice.

The eighth book is *Diet and Salad*, by N.W. Walker, available from O'Sullivan, Woodside and Company, 2218 East Magnolia, Phoenix, AZ 85034. The foods in this book to eat minimal amounts of are eggs, oil, dairy products, and honey. Also, there is too much emphasis placed on enemas, foot reflexology, and food combining.

The eight books described above will give you many creative ideas for healthful meal planning. Always remember to eat at least 75% (bulk, not calories) of your food uncooked. The number of different fruit and vegetable salads is so great that a raw food diet can be quite tasty and enjoyable. The improvement in health that will result is dramatic.

Following are recipes from the Center for Chiropractic and Conservative Therapy, 4310 Lichan Road, Penngrove, CA 94951.

« « « ◯ » » »

The center provides health care following the guidelines of this book including, but not limited to, supervised fasting.

For those not choosing a vegetarian diet, 4 to 5 ounces of poultry or fish can be added to one meal per day. Never fry these or any other foods.

Vegetable Salad

Any of the following ingredients can be included in whatever proportions you desire:

Grated carrot	Celery
Grated beet root (raw)	Cucumber
Grated or diced jicama root	Tomato
Cabbage (grated or sliced)	Avocado
Lettuce	Raw broccoli or cauliflower
Alfalfa (or other) sprouts	Raw sweet peas
Red or green bell pepper	or snow peas

Serving Suggestions: Serve with lemon wedges or natural salad dressing.

Individual Salad Bowls

Medium-sized pieces of lettuce (2 or 3 varieties)
Cut-up red cabbage
Sliced celery
Quartered tomatoes
Your choice of: sliced young tender zucchini or summer squash, a few small broccoli flowerets, a few snow peas or young tender green peas
Garnish with: pignolia nuts, sunflower seeds, and/or alfalfa sprouts

Serve with lemon juice or a blended avocado dressing.

Green Bean Salad

2 pounds fresh green beans, cut into 1 or 2 inch pieces
juice of 1 lemon
2 cloves garlic, finely minced
1/4 bunch parsley, minced
pinch basil

Cook the green beans in a skillet in a small amount of water until just tender. Drain and cool. Combine the beans with remaining ingredients. Chill and serve. Serves 4.

Asparagus Salad

2 lb. fresh asparagus (or substitute frozen)
4 oz. raw pumpkin seeds (pepitas; or substitute
    chopped almonds)
4 leaves Romaine lettuce
2 large or 4 small tomatoes
1 large or 2 small stalks bok choy
1 grapefruit (optional)

Asparagus may be used either raw or cooked or a combination of the two. If you use it raw, use only the tasty tender tips. If you use the asparagus cooked, cut off the very tough and discolored bottom ends of the stalks and steam the tender ends for 2 to 3 minutes, taking care not to overcook. You may use the tender tips raw and then steam the more fibrous (but not tough) portions and use both in your salad.

Cut up asparagus and place in a large mixing bowl along with pumpkin seeds.

Wash, dry, and cut or break up Romaine lettuce into bowl; wash and cut up tomatoes into bowl. If your tomatoes are not very tasty, you may wish to halve and juice a grapefruit and add the juice to your salad.

Wash celery and bok choy, dice coarsely, and add.

Mix well and then chop up with a paring knife to further blend ingredients. Serves 2.

Nutty Broccoli Salad

Broccoli
Celery
Cherry tomatoes
Pignolias
Pecans
Lemon juice

Wash and cut up broccoli and celery (use twice as much broccoli as celery). Wash and halve a fairly large quantity of cherry tomatoes. Chop pecans and juice about 1/2 lemon for every two people being served. Place all ingredients in a large bowl and mix well.

Serving suggestions: Alfalfa and other sprouts can be placed on top of each serving if desired. This salad can be eaten as is or served with a plateful of washed whole lettuce leaves for making lettuce sandwiches.

Cauliflower Salad

1 cauliflower, cut into flowerets
1 carrot, thinly sliced
1 green pepper, diced
1/2 cup lemon juice or juice of 1 lemon
1 clove garlic, minced (optional)
1/2 bunch parsley, minced
3 green onions, thinly sliced

Place the cauliflower, carrot, and green pepper in a steamer basket or a pot with a little water and steam covered for three minutes. Drain and cool, then transfer to a salad bowl.

Combine the lemon juice or vinegar, garlic, parsley, and green onions, and pour over the vegetables, tossing gently to distribute dressing. Chill and serve.

Serves 4.

Chinese Cabbage Salad

8 leaves Chinese cabbage
2 red bell peppers
2 avocados
1 pint cherry tomatoes (or 3 regular tomatoes)
1 grapefruit

Wash and dry Chinese cabbage; cut up four of the leaves and place in a large mixing bowl. Place remaining four leaves on two dinner plates. Wash and dice red bell peppers; quarter, peel, and dice avocados (or halve avocados and scoop out flesh with a teaspoon). Place peppers and avocados, along with washed and halved (or diced) tomatoes in mixing bowl.

Juice grapefruit and pour juice over ingredients in mixing bowl. Stir well and place a dollop of salad on each of the four Chinese cabbage leaves on the dinner plates. Serve remaining salad in bowls. Serves 2.

Eggplant Salad

1 eggplant
3 to 4 tomatoes
1 stalk celery
1 avocado (optional)
Lettuce or sprouts

Peel and dice eggplant into bite-sized chunks; place on a steamer in a pan with about 1 1/2 inches of water in it. With the lid on, start it steaming on high heat. Then turn the heat very low and steam for about 5 minutes.

Place steamed eggplant in a large bowl with washed and cut-up tomatoes. Wash and cut up broccoli and celery and mix with tomatoes and steamed eggplant chunks in a large bowl.

A diced avocado may be added to make this a main-course salad. Serve on beds of lettuce on plates or in bowls lined with lettuce or sprouts. Serves 2.

Eggplant Parmigiana

2 medium eggplants
8 oz. cashews
3 medium tomatoes
2 stalks celery
1 red (or green) bell pepper

Peel eggplants, slice 3/4 inch thick, and steam 6 to 8 minutes on low heat (after bringing to a steam on high heat).

Grind cashews in a blender or nut and seed grinder; place in a bowl and set aside.

Make fresh tomato sauce (see recipe page 186); slice tomatoes (circular slices); dice celery and pepper.

Place steamed eggplant slices on serving plates and layer on sliced tomatoes, diced celery and pepper, and ground cashews. Add another layer of sliced and diced veggies and ground cashews and serve.

Serves 2.

Eggplant with Tomato Sauce

1 eggplant, diced
10 to 12 large ripe tomatoes (or 12 oz. unsalted tomato paste)
1 large bell pepper, diced
8 to 10 mushrooms, sliced
Small amount green onion, leek, or chives (optional)
Basil and/or oregano to taste

Cut tomatoes into a large saucepan over low heat. Cover and heat for 3 to 5 minutes until tomatoes begin to soften. Add bell pepper, mushrooms, onion, herbs and diced eggplant. Mixture should be the consistency of thick soup. It may be necessary to add a small amount of distilled water or a few tomatoes or a little tomato paste in order to get the desired consistency.

Cook over low heat approx. 30 minutes. Cooking time may vary depending on size of eggplant chunks and temperature of low setting. Stir frequently while cooking.

Serve with brown rice or other grain, or over baked potatoes. Serves 4 to 6.

Butternut Corn Hotpot

4 cobs young sweet corn
1 to 1 1/2 pounds butternut pumpkin
3 medium carrots, scrubbed
1 pound fresh peas in pod
2 tablespoons chopped chives
4 to 6 ounces fresh mushrooms, diced
1/4 teaspoon ground ginger

Preheat oven to 300°.

Steam the corn cobs until the kernels are tender (about 15 minutes). Remove the corn, cut the corn kernels from the cobs, taking care to remove the entire kernel, especially the tiny germ at the head. Put the kernels in a small bowl and mix them with the chives.

Meanwhile, steam the pumpkin, carrots, and peas in their pods. When they just become tender, remove them from the steamer.

Saute mushrooms and ginger in 1 to 2 tablespoons of water for 5 minutes. (Chives or green onions are optional here.)

Cut the skin from the pumpkin and dice or slice as preferred. Slice the carrots and remove the peas from their pods.

Place layers of vegetables into a casserole dish, with corn mixture forming a center layer and the mushroom mixture poured over top. Cover the casserole dish and put it in the oven until the casserole is thoroughly heated through (about 15 minutes). Serves 4.

Tangy Avocado Dressing

2 medium avocados
1 tablespoon fresh lemon juice
1 tablespoon fresh chives, chopped

Peel, stone, and dice avocados. Put all the ingredients into a shallow mixing bowl, and mash them until smooth. Serve with a large salad.

Pecan Dressing or Dip

Shelled pecans
Fresh tomatoes

Grind up pecans. Wash and quarter tomatoes (or use whole cherry tomatoes) and place tomatoes in blender. Liquefy tomatoes and then add pecans. Blend on high speed, adding more tomatoes or pecan meal as needed to obtain desired thickness.

Use as a dressing for vegetable salads or as a dip for vegetables such as celery, broccoli, lettuce leaves, cauliflower, etc.

Carrot Deluxe

6 carrots, thinly sliced
2 apples, peeled and cut into chunks
1 tablespoon frozen apple juice concentrate
Juice of 1 lemon
1/2 teaspoon cinnamon

Mix all the ingredients and chill before serving. Serves 6.

Baked French Fries

Potatoes, preferably organic

Preheat oven to 450°.
Steam washed whole potatoes until just done (15–20 minutes for medium-small potatoes). Allow to cool on a plate, cutting board, or rack.
Slice potatoes into desired size and shape, place on a cookie sheet, and bake until crispy.

Lentils with Vegetables

2 cups dry lentils
4 to 6 cups distilled water
2 carrots, diced
2 stalks celery, diced
2 medium tomatoes, diced
Small amount of diced green onion, leek, or chives, if
    desired
Oregano or other herbs to taste

Bring 4 cups of water to a boil. Add lentils, cover, and turn to low setting. Allow lentils to cook for approx. 30 minutes, checking water level frequently. It may be necessary to add water as lentils swell.

Add vegetables and continue cooking 15 to 20 minutes on low temperature, stirring frequently; add water if necessary. If mixture is too watery, cook with cover off. Mixture should be thick and soupy.

Serve with brown rice, over baked potato, or on corn tortillas which have been crisped in an oven. Alfalfa sprouts, avocado, and fresh tomato may be layered on top to make a tostada. Serves 4 to 6.

Lentil Casserole

Lentil sprouts
1/2 lemon
1 medium tomato
2 stalks celery
1 medium avocado

Pour sprouted lentils into salad bowls.

Juice lemon half and place in blender, along with washed and quartered tomato, and liquefy on high speed. Wash celery, cut off leaves, cut into sixths, and gradually add through opening in blender lid while blender is running on high speed.

Quarter, peel, and add avocado to running blender and liquefy until smooth and creamy. Pour avocado-tomato sauce over lentil sprouts, mix well, and serve. Serves 2.

Vegetable-Nut Casserole

1/4 medium green cabbage, coarsely shredded
1/4 medium red cabbage, coarsely shredded
1/2 small cauliflower, broken into flowerets
2 medium carrots, thinly sliced
1 large pepper, preferably red, cored and diced
2 medium artichokes, halved and sliced (retain the core)
6 to 8 oz. ground seeds or nuts

Preheat oven to 175°.

Wash all the vegetables and place them in a large casserole dish and mix. Cover the dish and place in the oven. Cook until just tender (about 30 minutes, slightly longer if a deep dish is used).

Serve hot. Serves 6.

Garden Vegetable Mix

2 large stalks broccoli (chop stems and cut heads into
    flowerets)
2 carrots, sliced
2 tomatoes, quartered
2 stalks celery, sliced
1 green pepper, sliced into rings
1/4 head cauliflower, cut into flowerets
12 green beans, broken in half, with the ends removed
1/2 bunch parsley, finely chopped
Juice of 1/2 lemon (optional)

Place all the ingredients except the lemon juice in a large pot; add 3 cups water. Bring to a boil, lower heat, cover, and simmer over low heat for about 15 minutes. If desired, add the lemon juice before serving.

Serves 4.

Note: This preparation results in very tender vegetables and a relatively large amount of leftover cooking liquid, which may be enjoyed as a broth or reserved for use in other recipes as a vegetable stock.

Baked Vegetables

Potatoes, yams, and winter squash or pumpkins may be baked by placing in an oven and heated to 375 to 400°. Potatoes and yams should be pricked with a fork before baking. Yams and squash may be wrapped in aluminum foil to prevent dripping in the oven. Test periodically with a fork to determine if vegetables are done. Time varies with size of vegetables and temperature of oven. Squashes may be cut into smaller pieces to shorten cooking time.

Chinese Vegetables

1/2 cup water or vegetable stock
4 cups chopped bok choy
4 cups bean sprouts
1/2 cup tomatoes, quartered
1/2 to 1 teaspoon powdered ginger
1/2 teaspoon garlic powder
1/2 teaspoon onion powder

Heat the water or stock in a large skillet. Add the bok choy and cook over moderate heat, stirring occasionally. After about 5 minutes, add the bean sprouts, tomatoes, snow peas, and seasonings. Continue to cook, stirring as necessary, until the vegetables are tender. Serves 4.

Cauliflower Combination

1 head cauliflower, broken into flowerets
1 clove garlic, mashed (optional)
1 slice ginger, the size of a quarter, minced
1 yellow squash, cut into 1/2 inch pieces
1 red or green bell pepper, cut into 1/4 inch strips
3 tomatoes, cut into wedges
1/2 teaspoon oregano
1/2 teaspoon basil
1/2 cup green peas, fresh or frozen

Precook the cauliflower in a covered steamer basket or in a pot with a little water until partially cooked. Drain the cauliflower and reserve the cooking liquid. In a large skillet, saute the garlic and ginger for 1 minute in a few tablespoons of water. Add the cauliflower and a few tablespoons of the reserved cooking liquid and stir-fry the cauliflower for 2 minutes. Add the squash, peppers, and a few more tablespoons of the reserved cooking liquid if necessary and stir-fry for 2 more minutes. Add the tomatoes, seasonings, and about 1/2 cup of the reserved cooking liquid and cover and steam for 5 minutes. Remove the cover, add the peas, and cook for 3 to 4 minutes or until vegetables are tender. Serves 8.

Steamed Vegetables

Place stainless steel steamer basket in large saucepan and add water to within 1/4 inch of bottom of basket. Wash and cut vegetables into desired sizes and place in steamer basket. Bring water to a boil and allow vegetable to cook. Check frequently with a fork and remove vegetables promptly when done to avoid overcooking. It is best to put vegetables which require longer cooking time (corn, carrots, etc.) in first and add less dense vegetables later if you wish to have everything done at the same time.

Vegetable Sushi

Romaine lettuce
Chinese cabbage
Red bell pepper
Avocado
Nori

Wrap a peeled avocado quarter and a washed red pepper half in nori. Wrap a washed cabbage leaf around the avocado, pepper and nori, making the fold opposite the nori fold. Finally, wrap a washed lettuce leaf around the whole thing, folding on one of the open sides.

Potato Casserole

6 medium potatoes
2 medium sweet potatoes, preferably red
1 large eggplant
4 medium zucchinis
2 medium carrots
2 stalks celery, diced
4 to 6 oz. fresh mushrooms, washed and sliced
2 tablespoons water

Preheat oven to 330°.

Cut potatoes and sweet potatoes lengthwise, then slice them about 1/8" thick; do not peel. Thinly peel eggplant; cut it into four lengthwise, then slice it in about 1/4" thick pieces. Slice zucchinis about 1/2" thick. Slice carrots about 1/8" thick.

Arrange in layers half the prepared potato, sweet potato, eggplant, zucchini, and carrot. Sprinkle half the celery and mushroom over the top, and then repeat the layers. Add 2 tablespoons water to casserole dish.

Cover the casserole and place in oven until vegetables are tender (about 1 3/4 hours). Serves 4.

Brown Rice

2 cups long or short grain brown rice
4 cups water

Bring water to a boil. Add rice; turn heat to low. Cover and allow to cook approximately 40 minutes until water is absorbed.

Baked Tomatoes

3 large tomatoes, halved
2 tablespoons dried parsley
2 tablespoons minced chives (optional)
1 tablespoon basil
2 tablespoons grated almonds

Place the halved tomatoes cut side up in a shallow nonstick baking pan. Sprinkle the parsley, chives, basil, and almonds over the tomatoes. Bake at 325° until tender, about 15 to 20 minutes.
Serves 6.

Tasty Vegetarian "Tacos"

Whole lettuce leaves (Boston, Romaine, Bibb, or Leaf)
Creamy ripe avocados
Tomatoes (add lemon juice if you can't get tasty tomatoes)
Cilantro (a relative of parsley)
Alfalfa sprouts
Special Taco Sauce (see recipe below)

Wash and dry lettuce leaves and place on a platter.

Quarter and peel avocados; slice each quarter lengthwise twice; place avocado slices on a plate. With tomatoes sitting stem up, wash and cut into 1/2 inch strips and place on a plate. If you use lemon juice in addition to tomatoes, simply cut lemon into wedges and place on a plate. (Or you may juice lemons and place lemon juice in a small pitcher).

Wash cilantro, removing bad leaves; cut off roots; place on cutting board; cut up finely and put in a bowl. Serve alfalfa sprouts in a bowl also, and serve generous portions of Special Taco Sauce to each individual in cups or small bowls.

To assemble, place a lettuce leaf on a large plate; then fill the center, lengthwise, with avocado strips, tomato strips (and lemon juice), cut-up cilantro, taco sauce, alfalfa sprouts; and fold each side of the lettuce leaf over, and eat with your hands.

Special Vegetarian "Taco" Sauce

Shelled pecans
Tomatoes
Grapefruit
Lemon
Celery

Wash and quarter tomatoes and place in blender, along with juiced grapefruit (1/2 for every one or two persons) and lemon (1/4 per person). Liquefy tomatoes in citrus juices on highest blender speed; wash celery, cut off leaves and cut into sixths; and, with blender running, gradually add celery through opening in blender lid, blending until liquefied. If too acid or too bland, add more celery to suit taste.

Then, with blender running on high speed, add pecans through opening in blender lid. When mixture become too thick to blend, stop and start blender to get it going again. When that doesn't work, stop blender and stir contents before blending again, repeating as often as necessary. With blender stopped, stir in more tomato if more liquid is needed.

Ratatouille

1/2 cup water or vegetable stock
1 cup cubed eggplant
1 cup diced tomatoes
1 clove garlic, minced (optional)
1 teaspoon fresh oregano or 1/2 teaspoon dried oregano
1 teaspoon fresh basil or 1/2 teaspoon dried basil
1 cup diced celery
1 cup finely chopped green pepper
2/3 cup thinly sliced zucchini
2/3 cup diced mushrooms
Sauce:
1 cup tomato sauce
1 tablespoon frozen apple juice concentrate
1 tablespoon lemon juice
1 tablespoon cornstarch

In a skillet, saute the eggplant, tomatoes, garlic, and herbs together in the stock or water until the eggplant is 1/4 done. Add the other vegetables and cook until almost done.

Using a wire whisk, combine the sauce ingredients and pour over the vegetables. Mix well and cook, covered, until slightly thickened.
Serves 4.

Spaghetti Squash "Pasta"

1 large spaghetti squash (about 5 pounds)
8 sprigs parsley
Sauce:
Two 29 oz. cans tomato sauce (unsalted)
4 cups water
1 clove garlic, minced
1 1/2 teaspoons oregano
1 1/2 teaspoons basil

Combine all the sauce ingredients in a large saucepan. Bring to a boil, then reduce the heat and simmer uncovered for at least 2 hours.

Cut the squash in half with a heavy knife. (The squash can be cut crosswise or lengthwise: cutting it lengthwise produces longer strands.) Remove and discard the seeds. Place the squash halves, cut side down, in nonstick baking dishes. Bake at 350° for 1 hour, or until fork-tender. Using a fork, pull the cooked squash in strands from the skin.

Put 1 cup of the "spaghetti" on each plate. Pour 3/4 cup sauce over each serving (the sauce should be hot). Serves 8.

Artichokes with Fresh Tomato Sauce

4 medium artichokes
1 lemon, sliced
2 tablespoons chopped onions (optional)
6 cups chopped tomatoes (8 to 10 tomatoes,
    peeled if desired)
1/2 cup chopped parsley
1/4 cup lemon juice
1 teaspoon basil
1/2 teaspoon rosemary

Rinse the artichokes. Cut off the stems close to the base and cut 1 inch off the tops. In a large pot, bring 2 inches of water to boil and add the lemon slices and artichokes. Cover, turn down the heat, and simmer 25 to 30 minutes or until tender. Remove the artichokes from the pot, and turn upside down to drain.

Place the onion, garlic, and a few tablespoons of water in a large skillet and saute until the vegetables are soft. If the tomatoes are to be peeled, plunge them briefly in boiling water and then skin them. Stir in the chopped tomatoes and the remaining ingredients and simmer over low heat for 15 minutes, stirring occasionally.

Place the artichokes on individual serving dishes and spoon the tomato sauce around them. To eat, pull off a leaf, dip into sauce, and draw the fleshy portion off between the teeth; discard the remainder of the leaf. When you reach the center, remove the fuzzy section and eat the artichoke heart with sauce.

Variation: To make artichoke bowls to hold the tomato sauce, remove the center leaves and spread the artichokes open carefully. The fuzzy choke can be pulled out a little at a time, using a teaspoon (a serrated one works best) to remove the last bits. If desired, the bowls may be used to hold salads, jellied soups, or other sauces, or to hold dips for party buffets.

Fresh Tomato Sauce

> 5 medium tomatoes
> 1/2 lemon or lime, juiced
> 4 to 6 stalks celery
> 1 large or 2 small avocados

Wash and quarter tomatoes; place in blender along with lemon or lime juice; liquefy on highest blender speed.

Wash celery, cut off leaves, and cut into sixths. With blender running on high speed, gradually add celery and continue blending until celery is liquefied. If too acid or bland, add more celery to suit taste.

Peel, quarter, and add avocados; blend until smooth.

Fruit Pudding

In a blender combine bananas with any other sweet or subacid fruit. Serve immediately or keep very cold until served.

Apricot-Prune Whip

Soak overnight dried apricots and pitted prunes, and blend the next day with the soaking water. Serve plain or with sliced bananas.

Raw Apple Sauce

Wash, quarter, and core sweet juicy apples with skins on. Put in blender a few pieces at a time with a small amount of apple or lemon juice. Other fruits may be combined with the apples. Should be prepared immediately before serving, to keep color and flavor, or keep very cold until served.

Date Coconut Pie

Moisten fresh grated coconut with water and pat into pie plate for crust. Chill for an hour or so. Blend bananas and pitted dates in a little water (mixture should be quite thick) and pour over the crust. Put coconut liquid in blender and add small pieces of peeled coconut until you have a thick blended mixture, and spread over the pie. Top with shredded coconut and pitted dates, whole or sliced. Chill for at least 2 hours.

Frozen Seedless Grapes

Serve with toothpick handles.

Frozen Fruit Juice

Pour juice into ice cube trays and freeze. Serve with toothpick handles.

Banana Date Shake

Fresh fruit juice (apple, grape, or pear)
Frozen bananas
Dates

Peel and freeze bananas in plastic bag until hard. Pit dates (about two large or four small per serving). Make fresh fruit juice, either in a juicer or on the highest speed of a blender with a little distilled water. Next, on a high speed, blend dates with fruit juice. Then add frozen bananas, 1/2 or 1/3 at a time, and continue blending. This creamy-smooth drink is a meal in itself.

Apricot Banana Shake

Dried and/or fresh apricots
Distilled water
Peeled and frozen bananas
Dates

Peel ripe bananas and freeze in plastic bags until firm. Soak dried apricots several hours or overnight in enough water to cover them. Then blend them with the soaking water on high speed along with fresh apricots if available.

Add one to three pitted dates per serving and continue blending. Then add frozen bananas, a half banana at a time, blending until thick, smooth, and creamy.

Serve immediately.

Frozen Banana Delight

Ripe bananas

Peel ripe bananas; place in a single layer in plastic bags; secure with twisties; freeze overnight (or several hours).

At least 15 minutes before making, assemble juicer parts so the blank (not the screen) is in place, and put assembled parts and juicer blade in freezer (so the first banana you put through the juicer won't come out melted.).

Make *immediately* before eating it. (Do not store in freezer.) Put juicer blade and attachment on juicer and place a bowl at end of attachment. Remove frozen bananas from freezer; break bananas in half; and feed through juicer. Out comes a rich, creamy, frozen custard!

BIBLIOGRAPHY

Chapter 3: What is Health?

Dorland's Medical Dictionary, 25th Edition, 1974. W.B. Saunders Co., Philadelphia.

Shelton, Herbert M. 1928. *Human Life—Its Philosophy and Laws.* How To Live Publishing Co., Oklahoma City. Reprinted by Health Research Co., Mokelumne Hill, Calif.

Chapter 4: Health Philosophy

Webster's New World Dictionary, 1960. World Publishing Co., Cleveland.

Contact the American Natural Hygiene Society, 12816 Race Track Rd., Tampa, FL 33625, (813) 855-6607 for a comprehensive list of books and cassette tapes on this subject.

Chapter 5: Toxemia

Bjorksten, Johan, 1958. "A Common Molecular Basis for the Aging Syndrome," *Journal of the American Geriatric Society*, 6:740-748.

_____. 1968. "The Crosslinkage Theory of Aging." *Journal of the American Geriatric Society*, 16:408-427.

Tilden, John H., M.D. *Toxemia—The Basic Cause of Disease.* Natural Hygiene Press, Tampa, FL. Written in early 1900s, reprinted in 1974.

References linking minimal food intake with anti-aging can be found under Chapter 13 below.

References linking cholesterol and homocystine with heart disease can be found under Chapter 8 below.

Chapter 6: Inflammation

Robbins, Stanley L, M.D., and Ramzi S. Cotran, M.D. 1979. *Pathologic Basis of Disease*, 2nd edition. pp. 55-56. W.B. Saunders Co., Philadelphia.

Chapter 7: Progression of Pathology

Allen, Hannah. 1977. *Are You A Candidate For Cancer?* 2nd edition. Natural Hygiene Press, Tampa, FL.

Dorland's Medical Dictionary, op. cit.

Chapter 8: Heart Disease and Strokes

Consensus Development Conference Statement, 1984. "Lowering Blood Cholesterol to Prevent Heart Disease," Dec. 10-12. NHLBI Information Office, 9000 Rockville Pike, Building 31, Room 4A21, Bethesda, MD 20205.

Ende, N. 1962. "Starvation Studies with Special Reference to Cholesterol." *American Journal of Clinical Nutrition.* 11:270-280.

Enos, W.F., Major, et. al. 1953. "Coronary Disease among United States Soldiers Killed in Action in Korea," *Journal of the American Medical Association,* 152:1090-1093.

Hartung, G.H., et. al. 1980. "Relation of Diet to High Density Lipoprotein Cholesterol in Middle-Aged Marathon Runners, Joggers, and Inactive Men." *New England Journal of Medicine.* 302:357-361.

Jagannathan, S.N., et. al. 1974. "The Turnover of Cholesterol in Human Atherosclerotic Arteries," *Journal of Clinical Investigation,* 54:366-377.

Keys, A. 1967. "Dietary Factors in Atherosclerosis," *Cowdry's Arteriosclerosis,* H.T. Blumenthal, Editor, Charles C. Thomas, Springfield, IL. p. 585.

Kokatnur, M.G., et. al. 1975. "Depletion of Aortic Free and Ester Cholesterol by Dietary Means in Rhesus Monkeys with Fatty Streaks." *Atherosclerosis,* 21:195-203.

Malmros, H. 1950. "The Relation of Nutrition to Health." *Acta Medica Scandinavia.* 246 (supplement):137-153.

Morris, J.N., et. al. 1973. "Vigorous Exercise in Leisure Time and the Incidence of Coronary Heart Disease." *Lancet* 1:333-339.

Orten, J.M., and O.W. Newhaus. 1975. *Human Biochemistry,* 9th edition. C.V. Mosby Co., St. Louis. p. 285.

Pelletier, K.R. 1977. *Mind As Healer, Mind As Slayer.* Dell Publishing Co., New York.

Ross, R. and J.A. Glomset, M.D. 1976. "The Pathogenesis of Atherosclerosis." *New England Journal of Medicine,* 295:369-375.

Strom, A., and R.A. Jensen. 1951. "Mortality from Circulatory Diseases in Norway, 1940-1945." *Lancet* 1:126-129.

Thorn, G.W., et. al. 1977. *Harrison's Principles of Internal Medicine,* 8th edition. McGraw-Hill Book Co., New York.

Wilens, S.L. 1947. "The Resorption of Arterial Atheromatous Deposits in Wasting Disease," *American Journal of Pathology,* 23:793-804.

Chapter 9: High Blood Pressure

Boyer, J.L., and F.W. Kasch. 1970. "Exercise Therapy in Hypertensive Men," *Journal of the American Medical Association,* 211:1668.

"1979 Build and Blood Pressure Study." Ad Hoc Committee of the New Build and Blood Pressure Study. Association of Life Insurance Medical Directors of America and Society of Actuaries.

Choquette, G., and R.J. Ferguson. 1973. "Blood Pressure Reduction in 'Borderline' Hypertensives Following Physical Training," _Journal of the Canadian Medicine Association._ 108:699.

Duncan, G.G., et. al. 1964. "The Control of Obesity by Intermittent Fasts," _Medical Clinics of North America,_ 48:1359-1372.

Meneely, G.R., and H.D. Battarbee. 1976. "High Sodium-Low Potassium Environment and Hypertension," _American Journal of Cardiology._ 38:768.

Patel, C.H. 1973. "Yoga and Biofeedback in the Management of Hypertension," _Lancet_ 2:1053.

_____. 1975. "12 Month Follow-up of Yoga and Biofeedback in the Management of Hypertension," _Lancet_ 1:62.

Physicians' Desk Reference, 39th edition. 1985. Medical Economics Publishing Co., Ordell, NJ.

Reisin, E., et. al. 1978. "Effect of Weight Loss without Salt Restriction on the Reduction of Blood Pressure in Overweight Hypertensive Patients." _New England Journal of Medicine._ 298:1.

Chapter 10: Cancer

Brown, R.R. 1983. "The Role of Diet in Cancer Causation." _Food Technology,_ 37:49.

Carroll, K.K. 1975. "Experimental Evidence of Dietary Factors and Hormone-Dependent Cancers." _Cancer Research_ 35:3374-3383.

Epstein, S.S. 1974. "Environmental Determinants of Human Cancer." _Cancer Research,_ 34:2425-2435.

Herbert, Victor, M.D. 1979. "Laetrile: The Cult of Cyanide. Promoting Poison for Profit." _American Journal of Clinical Nutrition._ 32:1121-1158.

National Research Council, 1982. _Diet, Nutrition, and Cancer._ National Academy Press, Washington D.C.

Pearce, M.L., and S. Dayton. 1971. "Incidence of Cancer in Men on a Diet High in Polyunsaturated Fat." _Lancet_ 1:464-467.

Pinckney, E.R., M.D. 1973. "The Potential Toxicity of Excessive Polyunsaturates," _American Heart Journal_ 85:723-726.

Prehn, R.T. 1964. "A Clonal Selection Theory of Chemical Carcinogenesis." _Journal of the National Cancer Institute._ 32:1-15.

Ross, M.H., and G. Bras. 1971. "Lasting Influence of Early Caloric Restriction on Prevalence of Neoplasms in the Rat." _Journal of the National Cancer Institute._ 47:1095-1113.

Visek, W.J. et.al. 1978. "Nutrition and Experimental Carcinogenesis." *Cornell Veterinarian,* 68:3-39.

Warburg, Otto. 1956. "On the Origin of Cancer Cells." *Science* 123:309-314.

Wynder, E.L, and G.B. Gori. 1977. "Contribution of the Environment to Cancer Incidence: An Epidemiologic Exercise." *Journal of the National Cancer Institute* 58:825-832.

Chapter 11: Diabetes

Barnard, R.J., et. al. 1982. "Response of Non-Insulin Dependent Diabetic Patients to an Intensive Program of Diet and Exercise." *Diabetes Care,* 5:370-374.

Crapo, P.O., et.al. 1976. "Plasma Glucose and Insulin Responses to Orally Administered Simple and Complex Carbohydrates." *Diabetes* 25:741-747.

Genuth, S.M., M.D.. 1977. "Insulin Secretion in Obesity and Diabetes: An Illustrative Case." *Annals of Internal Medicine.* 87:714-716.

Jenkins, D.J.A, et.al. 1976. "Unabsorbable Carbohydrates and Diabetes: Decreased Post-Prandial Hyperglycemia," *Lancet,* July 24, 1976, pp. 172-174.

Kent, Saul. 1978. "Reevaluating the Dietary Treatment of Diabetes." *Geriatrics* 33:102.

Kiehm, T.G., et.al. 1976. "Beneficial Effects of a High Carbohydrate, High Fiber Diet on Hyperglycemic Diabetic Men." *American Journal of Clinical Nutrition* 29:895-899.

Miranda, P.M., et. al. 1978. "High Fiber Diets in the Treatment of Diabetes Mellitus." *Annals of Internal Medicine.* 88:482-486.

Stout, R.W., and J. Valance-Owen. 1969. "Insulin and Atheroma.." *Lancet* 1:1078-1080.

Thorn, G.W., et.al. *Harrison's Principles of Internal Medicine,* op. cit.

The University Group Diabetes Program. Diabetes 19 (Suppl. 2):747, 830, 1970. (Regarding oral diabetes drugs.)

Chapter 12: Hypoglycemia

Anderson, J.W., M.D., and R.H. Herman, M.D. 1975. "Effects of Carbohydrate Restriction on Glucose Tolerance of Normal Men and Reactive Hypoglycemic Patients." *American Journal of Clinical Nutrition.* 28:748-755.

O'Keefe, S.J.D., and V. Marks. 1977. "Lunchtime Gin and Tonic A Cause of Reactive Hypoglycemia." *Lancet,* June 18, pp. 1286-1288.

Thorn, G.W., et.al. *Harrison's Principles of Internal Medicine*, op. cit.

Chapter 13: Slowing the Aging Process

Barrows, C.H., and G.C. Kokkonen. 1977. "Relationship Between Nutrition and Aging." *Advances in Nutritional Research*, vol. 1, edited by H.H. Draper, Plenum Pub. Co., p. 253.

Dickerman, E., et.al. 1969. "Effects of Starvation on Plasma GH Activity, Pituitary GH, and GH-RF Levels in the Rat." *Endocrinology* 84:814.

"Dietary Preference, Growth, Aging, and Lifespan." 1977. *Nutrition Reviews* 35:49.

Everitt, A.V. 1971. "Food Intake, Growth, and the Aging of Collagen in Rat Tail Tendon." *Gerontologia* 17:98.

Grossie, J., and C.W. Turner. 1962. "Thyroxine Secretion Rates During Food Restriction in Rats." *Proceedings of the Society for Experimental Biology and Medicine.* 110:631.

"Growth of Vegetarian Children." 1979. Editorial. *Nutrition Reviews* 37:108.

Hayflick, L. 1973. "The Biology of Human Aging." *American Journal of Medical Science* 265:432.

Holeckova, E., and M. Chvapil. 1965. "The Effect of Intermittent Feeding and Fasting and of Domestication on Biological Age in the Rat." *Gerontologia* 11:96.

Mann, G.V. 1974. "The Influence of Obesity on Health." *New England Journal of Medicine* 291:178 and 226.

Marks, H.H. 1960. "Influence of Obesity on Morbidity and Mortality." *Bulletin of the New York Academy of Medicine* 36:296.

McCay, D.M. 1947. "Effect of Retarded Feeding Upon Aging and Chronic Diseases in Rats and Dogs," *American Journal of Public Health* 37:521.

Ross, M.H. 1977. "Dietary Behavior and Longevity." *Nutrition Reviews* 35:257.

_____ and E. Lustbader. 1976 "Dietary Practices and Growth Responses as Predictors of Longevity." *Nature* 262:548.

Sheldrake, A.R. 1974. "The Aging, Growth, and Death of Cells." *Nature* 250:381.

USDA. 1963. *Composition of Foods*, Agriculture Handbook No. 8, United States Government Printing Office, Washington, DC.

Chapter 14: Osteoporosis

Recommended Dietary Allowances, 9th edition. 1980. Committee on Dietary Allowances, Food and Nutrition Board, National Research Council, National Academy of Sciences, Washington, DC.

Davis, G.K. 1959. "Effects of High Calcium Intakes on the Absorption of Other Nutrients." *Federation Proceedings* 18:1119-1124.

Forbes, R.M. 1960."Nutritional Interactions of Zinc and Calcium." *Federation Proceedings* 19:643-647.

Horowitz, M., et.al. 1984. "Effect of Calcium Supplementation on Urinary Hydroxyproline in Osteoporotic Postmenopausal Women." *American Journal of Clinical Nutrition* 39:857.

Huddleston, A.L., et.al. 1980. "Bone Mass in Lifetime Tennis Athletes." *Journal of the American Medical Association* 244:1107-1109.

Nilas, L. et.al. 1984. "Calcium Supplementation and Postmenopausal Bone Loss." *British Medical Journal* 289:1103.

Physician's Desk Reference, op. cit.

Sandstead, H.H. 1975. "Some Trace Elements which are essential for Human Nutrition: Zinc, Copper, Manganese, and Chromium." *Progress in Food and Nutrition Science* 1:371-391.

Chapter 15: Allergies and Asthma

Adverse Reactions to Foods, 1984. American Academy of Allergy and Immunology, Committee on Adverse Reactions to Foods, Natl. Inst. of Allergy and Infectious Diseases, U.S. Dept. Health and Human Services, Natl. Inst. of Health. pp. 123, 127, and 177.

Dickey, L.D., M.D. 1976. *Clinical Ecology.* Charles C. Thomas Pubishers, Springfield, IL

Physician's Desk Reference, op. cit.

Chapter 16: Infectious Diseases

Connor, W.E. 1979. "Too Little or Too Much: The Case for Preventive Nutrition." *American Journal of Clinical Nutrition* 32:1975.

Kluger, M.J. 1976. "The Importance of Being Feverish." *Natural History* 85:71.

Murray, M.J., and A. Murray. 1977. "Suppression of Infection by Famine and Its Activation by Refeeding, a Paradox?" *Perspectives in Biology and Medicine* 20:471.

Murray, M.J., et.al. 1979. "Anorexia of Infection as a Mechanism of Host Defense." *American Journal of Clinical Nutrition* 32:593.

Robbins, S.L, et.al. *Pathologic Basis of Disease,* op. cit.

Thorn, G.W. *Harrison's Principles of Internal Medicine,* op. cit. pp. 757-759.

Chapter 17: Arthritis

Coombs, R.R.A, et.al. 1981. "Early Rheumatoid-Like Joint Lesions in Rabbits Drinking Cows' Milk," *International Archives of Allergy and Applied Immunnology* 64:287.

Criep, L.H. 1946. "Allergy of Joints." *Journal of Bone Joint Surgery* 28:276.

DeVries, J. 1982. "British Doctor Says Food Allergy Can Produce Arthritis Symptoms." *Arizona Republic.* Aug. 1.

Dickey, L.D. *Clinical Ecology,* op. cit.

Good, R.A. 1981. "Nutrition and Immunity" *Journal of Clinical Immunology.* 1:3.

Houpt, J.B., et.al. 1973. "Tryptophan Metabolism in Man (With Special Reference to Rheumatoid Arthritis and Scleroderma)," *Seminars in Arthritis and Rheumatism* 2:333.

Little, C.H., et.al. 1983. "Platelet Serotonin Release in Rheumatoid Arthritis: A Study in Food-Intolerant Patients," *Lancet,* Aug. 6, p. 297.

Lucas, C.P., et.al. 1981. "Dietary Fat Aggravates Active Rheumatoid Arthritis," *Clinical Research* 29:754A.

Mandell, M. et.al. 1980. "The Role of Allergy in Arthritis, Rheumatism, and Associated Polysymptomatic Cerebro-viscero-somatic Disorders: A Double-Blind Provocation Test Study," *Annals of Allergy* 44:51.

Palmblad, J. et.al. 1977. "Acute Energy Deprivation in Man: Effect on Serum Immunoglobulins, Antibody Response, Complement Factors 3 and 4, Acute Phase Reactants, and Interferon-Producing Capacity of Blood Lymphocytes," *Clinical Experimental Immunology* 30:50.

Parke, A.L., et.al. 1981. "Rheumatoid Arthritis and Food: A Case Study," *British Medical Journal* 282:2027.

Silberberg, R., et.al. 1957. "Changes in Bones and Joints of Underfed Mice Bearing Anterior Hypophyseal Grafts." *Endocrinology* 60:67.

Simkin, P.A. 1976. "Oral Zinc Sulphate in Rheumatoid Arthritis," *Lancet,* Sept. 11, 1976. p. 539.

Skoldstam, L, et.al. 1979. "Effects of Fasting and Lactovegetarian Diet on Rheumatoid Arthritis." *Scandinavian Journal of Rheumatology* 8:249.

Stroud, R.M., et. al. 1980. "Comprehensive Environmental Control and Its Effect on Rheumatoid Arthritis." *Clinical Research* 28:791A.

Uden, Ann-Mari, et.al. 1983. "Neutrophil Functions and Clinical Performance after Total Fasting in Patients with Rheumatoid Arthritis." *Annals of Rheumatoid Diseases* 42:45.

Zeller, M. 1949. "Rheumatoid Arthritis-Food Allergy as a Factor," *Annals of Allergy* 7:200.

Chapter 18: Stomach and Intestinal Problems

Goodhart, R.S., and M.E. Shils. 1980. *Modern Nutrition in Health and Disease,* 6th Edition. Lea and Febiger, Philadelphia.

Jones, V. Alun, et. al. 1985. "Original Articles: Crohn's Disease: Maintenance of Remission by Diet." *Lancet,* no. 8448, vol. II., July 27, 1985, pp. 177-180.

Chapter 19: Skin Diseases
Guyton, A.C. 1976. *Textbook of Medical Physiology*, 5th Edition. W.B. Saunders Co., Philadelphia.

Chapter 20: Headaches
Berkow, R. 1977. *Merck Manual of Diagnosis and Therapy*, 13th Edition. Merck and Co., Inc., Rahway, NJ.
"Certain Foods Provoke Migraine." 1983. Editorial. *Nutrition Reviews* 41:41.
Egger, J., et. al. 1983. "Is Migraine Food Allergy? A Double-blind Controlled Trial of Oligoantigenic Diet Treatment." *Lancet*, Oct. 8, 1983, vol. II, p. 865.
Perkin, J.E., and J. Hartje. 1983. "Diet and Migraine: A Review of the Literature." *Journal of the American Dietetic Association* 83:459.

Chapter 22: How To Eat
Goodhart, R.S., and M.E. Shils. 1980. *Modern Nutrition in Health and Disease*, 6th edition. Lea and Febiger, Philadelphia.

Chapter 23: How Much Should We Eat?
American Natural Hygiene Society books and tapes, address above.
Dickey, Lawrence D. *Clinical Ecology*, op. cit.

Chapter 24: Protein
Allison, J.B. 1965. "The Concept and Significance of Labile and Overall Protein Reserves of the Body." *American Journal of Clinical Nutrition* 16:445.
Barrows, C.H. 1977. "Nutrition and Aging: The Time Has Come To Move from Laboratory Research to Clinical Studies." *Geriatrics*, March, 1977. p. 39.
Berlyne, G.M. 1968. "Dietary Treatment of Chronic Renal Failure." *American Journal of Clinical Nutrition* 21:547.
_____. 1967. "The Dietary Treatment of Acute Renal Failure." *Quarterly Journal of Medicine*, New Series, 36:59.
Carmena, R. 1972. "Dietary Management of Chronic Renal Failure." *Geriatrics* 27:95.
Chu, J-Y. 1975. "Studies in Calcium Metabolism—11 Effects of Low Calcium and Variable Protein Intake on Human Calcium Metabolism." *American Journal of Clinical Nutrition* 28:1028-1035.
Goodhart, R.S., et.al. *Modern Nutrition in Health and Disease*, op. cit.
Hegsted, D.M. 1952. "False Estimates of Adult Requirements." *Nutrition Reviews* 10:257.

Hegsted, D.M. 1968. "Minimum Protein Requirements of Adults." *American Journal of Clinical Nutrition* 21:352.

Kempner, W. 1948. "Treatment of Hypertensive Vascular Disease with Rice Diet." *American Journal of Medicine* 4:545.

Lappe, F.M. 1971. *Diet for a Small Planet.* Ballantine Books, NY.

McCully, K.S. 1969. "Vascular Pathology of Homosycteinemia: Implications for the Pathogenesis of Arteriosclerosis." *American Journal of Pathology* 56:111.

Recommended Dietary Allowances, op. cit.

Robinson, C.H. 1973. *Fundamentals of Normal Nutrition,* 2nd edition. MacMillan Pub. Co., New York.

Scrimshaw, N.S., et.al. 1966. "Protein Metabolism of Young Men During University Examinations." *American Journal of Clinical Nutrition* 18:321.

_____. 1966. "Effects of Sleep Deprivation and Reversal of Diurnal Activity of Protein Metabolism of Young Men," *American Journal of Clinical Nutrition.* 19:313.

Chapter 25: Fat

See chapters on Heart Disease and Strokes, and on Cancer for references linking dietary fat with these illnesses.

Consumer Reports. "It's Natural! It's Organic! Or Is It?" July 1980, volume 45, p. 410.

Goodhart, R.S., et.al., *Modern Nutrition in Health and Disease,* op. cit.

O'Gara, R.W., et.al. 1969. "Carcinogenicity of Heated Fats and Fat Fractions." *Journal of the National Cancer Institute* 42:275.

Williams, A.V., et.al. 1957. "Increased Blood Cell Agglutination Following Ingestion of Fat, A Factor Contribution to Cardiac Ischemia, Coronary Insufficiency, and Anginal Pain," *Angiology* 8:29.

Chapter 26: Carbohydrate

Burkitt, D.P. 1975. "Epidemiology and Etiology." *Journal of the American Medical Association* 231:517.

Cummings, J.H. 1973. "Progress Report—Dietary Fiber." *Gut* 14:69.

Goodhart, R.S., et.al. *Modern Nutrition in Health and Disease.* op.cit.

Haber, G.B., et.al. 1977. "Depletion and Disruption of Dietary Fiber—Effects on Satiety, Plasma-Glucose, and Serum-Insulin." *Lancet,* Oct. 1, p. 679.

Sanchez, A, et.al. 1973. "The Role of Sugars in Human Neutrophilic Phagocytosis." *American Journal of Clinical Nutrition* 26:1180.

Nutrition Society 31:331.

Chapter 27: Food Processing

Goodhart, R.S., et.al. *Modern Nutrition in Health and Disease,* op.cit. p. 497-505.

Harris, R.S., and E. Karmas. 1977. *Nutritional Evaluation of Food Processing,* 2nd edition. Avi Publishing Co., Westport, CT.

Pottenger, F.M. 1946. "The Effect of Heat-Processed Foods and Metabolized Vitamin D Milk on the Dentofacial Structures of Experimental Animals." *American Journal of Orthodontics and Oral Surgery* 32:467.

_____., et.al. 1939-1940. "Heat Labile Factors Necessary for the Proper Growth and Development of Cats." *Journal of the Laboratory for Clinical Medicine* 25:238.

Chapter 28: Fasting

American Natural Hygiene Society books and cassette tapes, address listed above.

Bloom, W.L. 1959. "Fasting as an Introduction to the Treatment of Obesity." *Metabolism* 8:214.

Cahill, G.F., and O.E. Owen. 1967. "Starvation and Survival." *Transactions of the American Clinical Climatological Association* 79:13. 1967.

Drenick, E.J., et.al. 1964. "Prolonged Starvation as Treatment for Severe Obesity." *Journal of the American Medical Association* 187:100.

Runcie, J. and T.E. Hilditch. 1974. "Energy Provision, Tissue Utilization, and Weight Loss in Prolonged Starvation." *British Medical Journal* 2:352, 1974.

_____. and V. Miller. 1966. "Treatment of Obesity by Total Fasting for up to 249 Days." *Lancet* 2:992.

Saudek, C.D. and P. Felig. 1976. "The Metabolic Events of Starvation." *American Journal of Medicine* 60:117.

Stewart, W.K., and L.W. Fleming. 1973. "Features of a Successful Therapeutic Fast of 382 Days' Duration." *Postgraduate Medical Journal* 49:203.

Chapter 29: Vegetarianism

Albert, M.J., et.al. 1980. "Vitamin B12 Synthesis by Human Small Intestine Bacteria." *Nature* 283:781.

Brown, P.T., and J.G. Bergan. 1975. "The Dietary Status of 'New' Vegetarians," *Journal of the American Dietetic Association* 67:455.

Editorial. 1980. *Journal of the American Dietetic Association* 77:61.

Ellis, F.R., and V.M.E. Montegriffo. 1970. "Veganism, Clinical Findings and Investigations." *American Journal of Clinical Nutrition* 23:249.

_____. and P. Mumford. 1967. "The Nutritional Status of Vegans and Vegetarians." *Proceedings, Nutrition Society* 26:205.

_____., et.al. 1976. "The Health of Vegans Compared with Omnivores: Assessment by Health Questionaire." *Plant Foods for Man* 2:43.

Hardinge, M.G., and F.J. Stare. 1954. "Nutritional Studies of Vegetarians, I. Nutritional, Physical, and Laboratory Studies." *Journal of Clinical Nutrition* 2:73.

_____, et.al. 1958. "Nutritional Studies of Vegetarians. III. Dietary Levels of Fiber." *American Journal of Clinical Nutrition* 6:523.

Immerman, Alan M. 1981. "Vitamin B12 Status on a Vegetarian Diet." *World Review of Nutrition & Dietetics* 37:38.

McKenzie, J. 1971. "Profile on Vegans." *Journal of Foods and Human Nutrition* 2:79.

Sanders, T.A.B., et.al. 1978. "Haematological Studies on Vegans." *British Journal of Nutrition* 40:9.

_____. 1978. "Studies of Vegans: The Fatty Acid Composition of Plasma Choline Phosphoglycerides, Erythrocythes, Adipose Tissue, and Breast Milk, and Some Indicators of Susceptibility to Ischemic Heart Disease in Vegans and Omnivore Controls." *American Journal of Clinical Nutrition* 31:805.

Smith, A.D.M. 1962. "Veganism: A Clinical Survey with Observations on Vitamin B12 Metabolism." *British Medical Journal* i:1655.

U.S. General Accounting Office. *Problems in Preventing the Marketing of Raw Meat and Poultry Containing Potentially Harmful Residues.* April, 1979.

Chapter 30: Vitamins and Minerals

Allaway W.H. 1975. "The Effect of Soils and Fertilizers on Human and Animals Nutrition." USDA Agriculture Bulletin 278, March.

Armstrong, R.W. 1964. "Environmental Factors Involved in Studying the Relationship between Soil Elements and Disease." *American Journal of Public Health* 54:1536.

Bonner, J. and J.E. Varner. 1965. *Plant Biochemistry.* Academic Press, New York.

Dinauer, R.C. 1972. "Micronutrients in Agriculture." Soil Science Society of America, Inc., Madison, WI.

USDA Miscellaneous Publication 664. 1948. "Factors Affecting the Nutritive Value of Foods."

Goodhart, R.S., et. al. *Modern Nutrition in Health and Disease,* op. cit.

Hamner, K.C., et.al. 1942. "Effect of Mineral Nutrition on the Ascorbic Acid Content of the Tomato." *Botanical Gazette,* 103:586.

Harris, R.S. et.al. *Nutritional Evaluation of Food Processing,* op. cit.

Levitt, J. 1969. *Introduction to Plant Physiology.* C.V. Mosby Co., St. Louis.

National Academy of Sciences. 1977. *Geochemistry and the Environment,* vol. II, Washington, D.C.

Schroeder, H.A. 1971. "Losses of Vitamins and Trace Minerals Resulting from Processing and Preservation of Foods." *American Journal Clinical Nutrition* 24:562.

Sheets, O. 1946. "Mississippi Agricultural Experimental Station Bulletin 437."

Chapter 31: To Supplement or Not

Bieri, J.G. 1973. "Effect of Excessive Vitamin C and E on Vitamin A Status." *American Journal of Clinical Nutrition* 26:382.

Briggs, M.H., et.al. 1973. "Urinary Oxalate and Vitamin C Supplements." *Lancet* 2:201.

_____. 1973. "Side Effects of Vitamin C." *Lancet* 2:1439.

_____. 1973. "Fertility and High-Dose Vitamin C." *Lancet* 2:1083.

_____. 1974. "Vitamin E Supplements and Fatigue." *New England Journal of Medicine.* 290:579.

Brown, R.G. 1973. "Possible Problems of Large Intakes of Ascorbic Acid." *Journal of the American Medical Association* 224:1529.

Christensen, N.A., et.al. 1964. "Hypercholestremia: Effects of Treatment with Nicotinic Acid for Three to Seven Years." *Diseases of the Chest* 46:411.

Corrigan, J.J., and F.I. Marcus. 1974. "Coagulopathy Associated with Vitamin E Ingestion." *Journal of the American Medical Association* 230:1300.

Dahl, S. 1974. "Vitamin E in Clinical Medicine." *Lancet* 1:465.

Dykes, M.H.M., and P. Meier. 1975. "Ascorbic Acid and the Common Cold—Evaluation of its Efficacy and Toxicity." *Journal of the American Medical Association* 231:1073.

Gershon, S.L, and I.H. Fox. 1974. "Pharmacologic Effects of Nicotinic Acid on Human Purine Metabolism." *Journal of Laboratory and Clinical Medicine* 84:179.

Hillman, R.W. 1957. "Tocopherol Excess in Man." *American Journal of Clinical Nutrition* 5:597.

Hunt, C.E., et.al. 1970. "Copper Deficiency in Chicks: Effects of Ascorbic Acid on Iron, Copper, Cytochrome Oxidase Activity, and Aortic Mucopolysaccharides." *British Journal of Nutrition* 24:607.

Lamden, M.P. 1971. "Dangers of Massive Vitamin C Intake." _New England Journal of Medicine_ 284:336.

Marx, W., et.al. 1949. "Effects of the Administration of a Vitamin E Concentrate and of Cholesterol and Bile Salt on the Aorta of the Rat." _Archives of Pathology_ 47:440.

Melhorn, D.K. 1969. "Relationships Between Iron-Dextran and Vitamin E in Iron Deficiency Anemia in Children." _Journal of Laboratory and Clinical Medicine_ 74:789.

Mosher, L.R. 1970. "Nicotinic Acid Side Effects and Toxicity: A Review." _American Journal of Psychiatry_ 126:9.

Patterson, J.W. 1950. "The Diabetogenic Effect of Dehydroascorbic and Dehydroisoascorbic Acids." _Journal of Biological Chemistry_ 183:81.

Stein, H.B., et.al. 1976. "Ascorbic Acid-Induced Uricosuria, A Consequence of Megavitamin Therapy." _Annals of Internal Medicine_ 84:385.

Shute, E. 1938. "Wheat Germ Oil Therapy." _American Journal of Obstetrics and Gynecology_ 35:249.

Telford, I.R. 1949. "The Effects of Hypo- and Hyper-Vitaminosis E on Lung Tumor Growth in Mice." _Annals of the New York Academy of Science_ 52:132.

Tsai, A.C., et.al. 1978. "Study on the Effect of Megavitamin E Supplementation in Man." _American Journal of Clinical Nutrition_ 31:831.

Udomratn, T., et.al. 1977. "Effects of Ascorbic Acid on Glucose-6-Phosphate Dehydrogenae-Deficient Erythrocytes: Studies in an Animal Model." _Blood_ 49:471.

Winter, S.L, and J.L. Boyer. 1973. "Hepatic Toxicity from Large Doses of Vitamin B3 (Nicotinamide)." _New England Journal of Medicine_ 289:1180.

Chapter 32: Calcium and Dairy Products
Recommended Dietary Allowances, op. cit.
Robinson, C.H. _Fundamentals of Normal Nutrition,_ op. cit.
Thorn, G.W., et.al. _Harrison's Principles of Internal Medicine,_ op. cit.
See chapter on Protein for further references.

Chapter 33: Feeding Babies
Marano, H. 1979. "Breast-Feeding: New Evidence It's Far More Than Nutrition." _Medical World News_ 20:62.

Smith, G.V., et.al. 1978. "Breast Feeding and Infant Nutrition." _American Family Physician_ 17:92.

Truesdell, D.D. and P.B. Acosta. 1985. "Feeding the Vegan Infant and Child." *Journal of the American Dietetic Association* 85:837.

Chapter 34: Herbs
Tyler, V.E. 1981. *The Honest Herbal* George F. Stickley, Philadelphia.

Chapter 35: Exercise
Bailey, C. 1978. *Fit or Fat?* Houghton Mifflin Co., Boston.
Crandall, D.L, et.al. 1981. "Relative Role of Caloric Restriction and Exercise Training upon Susceptibility to Isoproterenol-Induced Myocardial Infarction in Male Rats." *American Journal of Clinical Nutrition* 34:841.
Cooper, K.H. 1977. *Aerobics.* Bantam Books, New York.
Quig, D.W., et.al. 1983. "Effects of Short-Term Aerobic Conditioning and High Cholesterol Feeding on Plasma Total and Lipoprotein Cholesterol Levels in Sedentary Young Men." *American Journal of Clinical Nutrition* 38:825.
Shoenfield, Y. et.al. 1980. "Walking—A Method for Rapid Improvement of Physical Fitness." *Journal of the American Medical Association* 243:2062.
Simonelli, C., and R.P. Eaton. 1978. "Cardiovascular and Metabolic Effects of Exercise." *Postgraduate Medicine* 63:71.

Chapter 36: Stress
Benson, H. 1972. *The Relaxation Response.* Avon, New York.
Pelletier, K.R. 1977. *Mind as Healer, Mind as Slayer.* Dell Pub. Co., New York.

Chapter 37: Chiropractic
Altman, N. 1981. *The Chiropractic Alternative.* Houghton Mifflin Co., Boston.
Commission of Inquiry into Chiropractic. 1979. *Chiropractic in New Zealand.* Government Printer, Wellington.
Homewood, A.E. 1977. *The Neurodynamics of the Vertebral Subluxation.* Valkyrie Press, St. Petersburg.
Murray, Goldstein. *The Research Status of Spinal Manipulation Therapy.* U.S. Dept. of Health, Education and Welfare, Bethesda, MD.
Wilk, C.A. 1976. *Chiropractic Speaks Out.* Wilk Publishing Co., Park Ridge, Illinois.

Chapter 38: Drinking Water

Bagwell, K. 1985. "Valley TCE Pollution 'Tip of the Iceberg'." *Scottsdale Daily Progress,* July 2.

Begley, S., et.al. 1982. "How Safe is Your Water?" *Newsweek,* Nov. 1, p. 89.

Chicago Tribune. 1985. "Scientists Urge Steps to Curb Cancer Risk from Chemical's Use." Reprinted in *Arizona Republic,* Oct. 13. Regarding international meeting of scientists.

"Home Filters to 'Purify' Water." Feb., 1981. *Changing Times Magazine.* Regarding EPA study of water filters.

Maugh, T.H. 1981. "New Study Links Chlorination and Cancer." *Science* 211:694.

New York Times. 1982. "Report Details 'Serious' Threat to Ground Water." Reprinted in *Arizona Republic,* Dec. 29. Regarding EPA report on polluted surface water impoundments.

Perry, M.A.M. 1984. "Tainted Water is Sloshing under Valley." *Arizona Republic,* March 11.

United Press International. 1982. "EPA Considering Chemical Controls for Drinking Water." and "Foul Water is Causing Disease, Agency Says." *Arizona Republic,* March 7. Regarding GAO report on drinking water violations.

Wilkins, J.R., et.al. 1979. "Organic Chemical Contaminants in Drinking Water and Cancer." *American Journal of Epidemiology* 110:420.

Chapter 39: Rest and Sunshine

Brody, Jane E. *New York Times.* 1984. "Sun's Therapeutic Powers Praised, Studied." Reprinted in *Arizona Republic,* Nov. 14.

Shelton, Herbert M., op. cit.

Chapter 40: Diet and Menu Plans

Cinque, Ralph C., M.D. 1978. "Hygiene vs. USDA: Analysis of the Nutritional Quality of Two Diets." *Health Science Magazine,* vol. 1, no. 9, Dec. Published by ANHS. 12816 Race Track Rd., Tampa, FL 33625.

Goldhammer, Dr. Alan and Dr. Jennifer Marano. *A Rational Diet for Optimum Nutrition.* Center for Chiropractic and Conservative Therapy, Inc. 4310 Lichau Rd., Penngrove, CA 94951.

USDA Handbooks No. 8 and 456 on food composition.

RESOURCE DIRECTORY

Organizations:

1. American Natural Hygiene Society, P.O. Box 30630, Tampa, FL 33630. Write for a full listing of chapters and doctors; a few are mentioned below.
2. Natural Hygiene, Inc., P.O. Box 2132, Huntington Station, Shelton, CT 06484.
3. Canadian Natural Hygiene Society, P.O. Box 235, Station T, Toronto, Canada M6B 4A1.
4. Chicago Natural Hygiene Society, 202 Oxbow Ct., Valparaiso, Indiana 46383.
5. Phoenix Natural Hygiene Society, 5743 E. Thomas, Scottsdale, AZ 85251.
6. Life Science Institute, 6600 Burleson Rd., P.O. Box 17128, Austin, TX 78760.
7. Fit For Life (Diamonds), 2210 Wilshire Blvd., Suite 118, Santa Monica, CA 90403.

Doctors for Inpatient and Outpatient Care:

1. For a complete list, contact the ANHS (above).
2. Dr. Alan M. Immerman, 5743 E. Thomas Rd., Scottsdale, AZ 85251, (602) 946-1597.
3. Dr. Alan Goldhammer, 4310 Lichau Rd., Penngrove, CA 94951. (707) 792-2325.
4. Dr. Ralph Cinque, 439 East Main St., Yorktown, TX 78164. (512) 564-3670.
5. Dr. David Scott, P.O. Box 8919, Strongsville, OH (216) 238-6930.
6. Dr. John McDougall, St. Helena Hospital Health Center, Deer Park, CA 94576. (800) 862-7575.
7. Dr. William Esser, P.O. Box 6229, Lake Worth, FL 33466. (305) 965-4360.
8. Dr. Ron Cridland, Lobraico Ln., RR4, Stouffville, Ontario, Canada L4A 7X5.
9. Dr. Trevor Salloum, 557 Bernard Ave., Kelowna, British Columbia, Canada V1Y 6N9. (604) 763-5445.